Survivor's

Remorse

Survivor's Remorse

The Healing Power of Faith

Dr. Arthur D. Vaughn

Contents

More Than I Can Bear
7

Gracefully Broken
105

My Testimony
133

Appendix
191

More Than I Can Bear

1.

If we live, we live for the Lord; and if we die, we die for the Lord. So, whether we live or die, we belong to the Lord.

- Romans 14:8 New International Version (NIV)

It was the 4th of July, and my alarm went off at 5:00 a.m. I got prepared as it was time to get up and head to downtown Atlanta for the 50th Peachtree Road Race (the Peachtree), which was my eighth straight race. I have trained tirelessly for this day and was looking forward to completing this annual journey. Like the other 10,000 participants, I found a parking spot and headed to what was sure to be a crowded commuter train. As I joined the other walkers and runners, I made my way toward "group P" to catch up with a couple of my fraternity brothers. As usual, we took our obligatory photos, and the energy and excitement around this race became increasingly infectious the closer I got to the starting point! Now don't get me wrong, I was not in the competitive part of the race. I often say I run to complete, not to compete. I was aware I will be walking seventy-five percent of the race and would stop at every water station and at the top of "Cardiac Hill" where each year, I catch up with my good friend Chesley, a local meteorologist, to catch my breath, take a photo, and share a good laugh.

I felt really good about completing the race and was delighted to be out there. To get in sync with the race, I switched back and forth from the music playing through my earphones to listening to the disc jockeys. I saw my buddy, DJ MoHawk, at one station and got his attention — Mo and I have deejayed with local professional sports teams for the last twelve years. The race was always tough, as the heat and hills are brutal. After an hour and some minutes, I turned on to 10th street, running the last half-mile, and then sprint the final 100 meters or so. My body felt every step of the 6.2 miles, but what was important was the fact that I completed the race. Finally, I completed my eighth Peachtree and earned that coveted T-shirt.

I dragged myself through the park and stepped up to one of

the podiums in the park and took a photo with my arms raised in triumph. It turned out to be a good morning; I felt strong, vibrant, and accomplished. I didn't come in first by a long shot, but I felt great. My 50th birthday was just three months earlier, yet I was still participating in these races. I couldn't have been happier for myself!

During the drive home, the adrenaline from the race decreased and I gradually began to feel abnormally tired. Later, I learned that there was a good reason for this, which may have been the first warning sign of what is to come. Today, being the 4th of July, I just couldn't afford to miss the festivities that come with Independence Day. I also recognized that I haven't been around that much to spend time with my family, and as such, I did the needful by taking my wife to the Square for the fireworks. My daughters were already there spending time with their friends, and we figured we would catch up with them. I was struggling a bit, but I assumed it was just a result of the race, and I didn't place a lot of importance on how exhausted I felt.

The next day, I was scheduled to play a round of golf at a local course. Our foursome played nine holes and then it began to rain. So, we stopped at the clubhouse for lunch and then completed the back nine holes. I played with the accounting department chair at a local college and one of his buddies on their home course. They would often beat me at golf, so my loss that day was to be expected. As I think back, I have to admit that when I walk to the tee box and the green on holes seventeen and eighteen, I felt odd and a bit out of breath. I was winded, but again, I attributed it to having just run the Peachtree the day before. The rest of the weekend was all about family time. Usually, we would go to see the latest Marvel movie, run errands, and do stuff around the house. We don't do anything fancy, but we do it together.

2.

The Monday after the Peachtree rolled around, which happened to be the beginning of what became the worst month of my life. I headed back to work after a great 4-day weekend. I was working at my dream college, and while I Bleed Orange as a result of my time as a student at Syracuse University; the school I was working at was a solid second on my list of schools I wanted to attend coming out of high school. This single-gender African American male higher education institution I worked at is where I was meant to be. My calling was to work with young African American men to help them realize their highest aspirations. It had always been my dream to specifically work with young men who are not academically prepared for college but who, with a little tutoring and mentoring, would realize their dreams. Even though not all of the young men at this school were admitted with a profile that suggested additional support was needed, I wanted to help those who did. I believe this same passion has been the driving force for my service and mentoring with the 100 Black Men of America and Alpha Phi Alpha Fraternity, Inc. For me, being affiliated with the lore associated with the endless list of alumni and current students was like standing on top of a mountain. One of my friends often told me that I have more gear from the College than he did, and he actually graduated from the Institution. But let me be clear — I got my start at Syracuse University. LOL!

The Monday after the holiday weekend, I went to work feeling pretty good and ready for the week. My role at my workplace entails that I attend a lot of meetings, do a fair amount of financial analysis, and help others solve their fiscal issues. Midday came and we headed out for lunch. I walked down the same set of stairs I had walked up earlier to get to the 2nd-floor office, but the difference was that when I previously walked up to the office that morning, I felt fine and was in good condition. Due to the workload in the office, I began to run short of breath. Later the same day, I still wasn't recuperating and I mentioned my symptoms to my immediate supervisor, who then advised that I go straight to the hospital. Being the stubborn, macho person that I am, I insisted I stay for our 4 o'clock meeting. I convinced myself that it was just one more meeting and I had something to contribute to this important gathering of colleagues. After negotiating with my supervisor and human resources, we agreed that I would stay for the meeting but go home right after it ends.

When I arrived home, I was still having breathing issues but figured that we would find out what's going on the next day during my doctor's appointment. I wasn't sure why, but I grabbed my continuous positive airway pressure (C-PAP) machine, which helps me to breathe while sleeping due to my sleep apnea. Putting the C-PAP machine on became a surprising blessing because I needed the oxygen to aid my heart function. But I would have never known that — I just knew the C-PAP was helping me feel better. Cardiovascular disease poses the *greatest* health threat to Black Americans. The prevalence of high blood pressure (hypertension) in Black Americans is among the highest in the world, and it is rapidly increasing on a daily basis. A variety of factors influence this illness and are associated with health and longevity, which includes economic status, ethnicity, and access to care.

Dr. Arthur D. Vaughn

The next day, I kept the appointment to see my primary care physician, and after running the normal tests, he referred me to a cardiologist. I still think this is routine, so I casually said okay and suggested that he sends me back to the cardiologist I've seen before, Jonathan Patel, MD. Dr. Patel happened to be a friend and fraternity brother. I believe this relationship and trip to the doctor saved my life. In the past, I, like most men, would have tried to tough it out and not immediately call their physician or schedule the referral until after a week or two. As children and young adults, we are taught a masculine way of living that is needed to earn and maintain respect in the world. This façade, at its extreme, contributes to males seeking medical or mental health care less regularly. This negative notion of *"Be a Man" or "Man Up"* contributes to a culture that is killing us. One of the reasons I mention this is because the issues I am talking about may disproportionately affect Black and Brown men, but these issues are impacting men regardless of ethnicity or skin color.

We have to change the definition of the phrase, *Man Up*. Men are dying of heart disease at a rate two times higher than women (DHHS, 2020). To" Man Up" should be when we openly discuss our physical and mental health with one another in the same way we discuss the scores from last night's game. If we created safe spaces to discuss the daily pressures we face and the effects they have on us, I believe we would see decreases in the incidence of high blood pressure and heart disease in our community. I know this would be a radical change for many of us, but it would save lives.

3.

"He who did not spare his own Son, but gave him up for us all—how will he not also, along with him, graciously give us all things?"

- Romans 8:32, New International Version (NIV)

In retrospect, everything was falling into place through God's favor, grace, and mercy. As a child, I was taught that grace is God's love freely given to mankind. Experience tells me referrals to specialists can sometimes take days or weeks to schedule. As you will see later, every hour and day in my journey ended up being critical. During my visit with Dr. Patel, we again ran the normal tests, including computed tomography (CT), an echocardiogram (EKG), and a nuclear stress test. The tests the cardiologist ran are common as they are determinants in checking my heart function. At this point, I was still in denial, believing that nothing serious was going on and that I just needed to go through the motions.

Less than six minutes, after I was done exercising on the treadmill, I ran to the closest bathroom to vomit. It was at this point that I knew something was wrong. I ran the Peachtree and played golf less than a week ago, and days later, I can't jog for six minutes on a treadmill. My wife, Octavia, works a mile or two away from the doctor's office and I called her and asked her to come over. The staff wanted to perform a CT scan, but I hate tight places, and that tube they place patients in drives me crazy. Octavia also did not think anything major was going on at the time. She assured me that she would get me through being in an enclosed space, maybe hear the results and then return to work. The staff asked her to come back to where I was, and at first glance, she thought I looked weak, but assumed I was simply tired. At this time, we both expected Dr. Patel to tell us what they always say; "lose a little weight, exercise, change your diet, and take the pills I am going to prescribe." But he went straight in about the severity of my condition, explaining that I was suffering from acute heart failure with my heart function at twenty-five percent capacity. We learned that a healthy heart functions between fifty and seventy percent. My Ejection Fraction (EF) of twenty-five percent explained the shortness of breath and overall exhaustion I was experiencing.

"If you believe, you will receive whatever you ask for in prayer."

- Matthew 21:22 (NIV)

The doctor then shared with us that without a heart transplant, I was not likely to survive. Upon hearing the news, I fell to my knees and broke down sobbing and lamented, "I don't want to die, I don't want to die." My relaxed, carefree mood changed to one of despair and anger. He then shared that we needed to get me to the emergency room as soon as possible so I could be admitted. He also indicated that he would contact the hospital down the street in advance and a colleague would be waiting, so we could be ushered in immediately. Octavia was still in a bit of shock, as none of this seemed real to her. She thought she was coming to a routine doctor's appointment only to learn that I was dying. She asked Dr. Patel that if I was as thoroughly sick as he was saying, then why wasn't an ambulance called? His reply was that the hospital was literally across the street, and the time and effort to get them here would

21

be wasted versus driving the 1000 feet to the hospital. But he stressed that if we wanted to call an ambulance, then they would. We both remained in shock and questioned him further because this still didn't make sense, and we wondered if he was being dramatic or if I was really that ill. While a final diagnosis wasn't clear, he shared that there were definitely life changes that I needed to make and that I may need a transplant.

I was still in denial regarding what was going on, and I asked if I would have to give up smoking cigars — as if it would magically reverse my current situation. This was yet another indication that I was in disbelief as in the grand scheme of things. My habit of smoking cigars was inconsequential at this stage of my heart disease. Octavia challenged the doctor's suggestion that I wouldn't need to give up smoking and went as far as to say, "That's bullshit." She was firm in her belief then and believes now that smoking cigars is the same as cigarettes and is detrimental to heart function. We were both so far into our denial that we were more focused on cigars and not the real issue—I was in the middle of heart failure.

The doctor and Octavia agreed to disagree and returned the conversation to the need to get me to the hospital as quickly as possible. The staff then grabbed a wheelchair and took me to the car. After driving three feet, I asked that the car be pulled over and I vomited a second time. At this point, I believed the reason I became ill was as a result of nerves and the fear of death setting in, not the actual heart illness. The shock related to my being sick and the need for extreme measures were gradually taking over my mind and body. We were both in a mental space that showed we were out of touch with what was really going on. Denial is the first stage of grief and the time when people rationalize the situation and tell themselves, "This can't be happening to me when clearly that message is wrong" (Kübler-Ross & Kessler, 2005).

Later, through therapy, I started learning about coping mechanisms that people may find helpful when dealing with the type of denial I experienced. It was suggested that I learn about the disease and the procedures that I went through and continued to experience post-surgery. I would sit up at night with one of the nurses and go through my medical records and they would share with me what had happened and why it was needed. I also turned to the Internet to search for medical articles and peer-reviewed research to learn more about my illness. Since my health deteriorated so fast, I was only able to begin my research after surgery. Learning about all that

Dr. Arthur D. Vaughn

happened came with the display of emotion that is a mix of both joy and sadness.

4.

"Therefore we do not lose heart. Though outwardly we are wasting away, yet inwardly we are being renewed day by day."

- 2 Corinthians 4:16 (NIV)

Based on Dr. Patel's comments, we expected the hospital emergency department staff was aware that we were coming, but that wasn't the case at all. At the same time, I seemed to be further deteriorating; I was droopy, quiet, and lethargic. When we went to the check-in desk, they didn't seem to know why we were there and we sat and waited in the emergency room (ER) for thirty minutes until we were called by a staff who inquired to know why we were there. When we called Dr. Patel, he reached out to the physician that was supposed to meet us at the ER but to no avail. The ER staff's apparent laissez-faire attitude gave me the sense that they still need to register how serious my condition was. The ER staff eventually checked me in and began performing routine tests. Based on the results of the tests, the ER staff finally realized that I needed to be admitted to the hospital. I went from being in shock to being outright scared. I feared that I would not make it through the night. Although I was in prayer, my faith was shaken.

Shortly after being admitted, I began having chest pains and the providers called in a cardiac nurse. Within 30 minutes of being admitted, I was moved to the intensive care unit (ICU). After arriving in the ICU, additional monitors and probes were connected to stabilize my condition. I literally had tubes and wires sticking out of every part of my body.

A day later, the fun began! On Friday, July 12th, they took me to the operating room and a series of procedures were completed; a heart biopsy was performed, a pacemaker and a defibrillator were surgically implanted in my chest. The defibrillator is designed to shock a person's heart if they are about to go into cardiac arrest. These procedures are all typically done without full sedation and I was partially aware of everything that was going on. After returning from the operating room, I was more alert and talkative, yet still weak and as expected, mentally unable.

Over the next day or two, additional procedures had to be performed. While back in the operating room, the pressure around my heart was checked. A thin, flexible tube was inserted through my neck that ran into the left side of my heart to begin the diagnosis of the severity of the issue. The physicians determined that my heart suddenly couldn't pump enough blood to meet my body's needs, and a balloon pump was inserted in my left leg and a tube ran up next to my heart. The balloon pump is a mechanical device designed to increase the oxygen reaching one's heart and indirectly increases blood flow. The balloon was inserted into my aorta, which helped supply blood to my head, neck, shoulder, and arms. These were all very risky procedures and anyone of them could have resulted in my death. I didn't fully understand how dangerous these processes were until much later. Through all of this, I was comforted in my faith that this would work out but was also emotionally fragile while I attempted to hold it all together. All this bottled up emotion was not healthy and I needed to be comfortable releasing it as it was leading to other physical and emotional illnesses and trauma. This is when *Man Up* should mean being comfortable breaking down.

5.

"For I am the Lord your God who takes hold of your right hand and says to you, Do not fear; I will help you."

- Isaiah 41:13 (NIV)

After five days at St. Joseph's Hospital, my heart function dropped to nine percent. Having a heart function this low could be described as "sitting in a rowboat three-quarters full of water while frantically rowing across a big lake," says Dr. Patel. At this point, my heart was again unable to pump enough blood to tissues and organs to function. The medical interventions and drugs that sometimes had corrected my condition were simply not working. The physicians determined that a different level of care was needed, which led to my first helicopter ride. I was airlifted to Emory

University Hospital (Emory) and admitted to the Cardiovascular Intensive Care Unit (ICU).

I arrived at Emory while going in and out of consciousness and struggling to function. The transplant coordinator later confirmed the previous analogy, letting me know that I was the sickest of the sick, and while clinging to life through the use of machines, my heart was in complete failure. In an instant, my heartbeats-per-minute began to approach twice the normal rate in an attempt to compensate for my decreased heart function. Due to my failing heart, the fight against time was a battle of life and death.

My beats per minute rapidly increased and a pain that started in my right hand began to gradually move up my arm. The machines in the room started beeping and the lights began flashing at an increasingly rapid pace. All the motion around me was confusing and something I could not process at the moment; I was scared and without warning, my heart went into shock. The medical team initiated a flurry of activity to stabilize my heart function. All the calmness that was previously felt in the room turned into a sense of panic as the doctors began to rush in and started giving directions to each other using terms I couldn't understand, but it was too late. The defibrillator in my chest was triggered and it in turn shocked my heart, which lifted me out of bed, causing me to invent new combinations of curse words. I have never felt pain like that in my life and that was just the beginning.

My buddy, Eric, who was visiting with me at the time, was also caught off guard and literally fell out of the chair in surprise while trying to get out the way of the doctors. His movements were described to me as a combination of a crawl and a run to get out of the room. I later felt bad that he had to see this and the experience impacted him emotionally, as he felt he had just watched his friend die on the table.

After this episode, the cardiac care unit team was prepared and was able to manage the instances when I needed my heart shocked. Prior to being shocked, the sedation was designed to prevent me from being emotionally traumatized based on the experience, but I can tell you I was affected. I would hate to minimize the experience; even under partial sedation, this was an unbelievably frightening experience and each time was incredibly painful. The doctors provided me with oxygen to regulate my breathing as I began to go into convulsions. It took approximately 30 minutes before I became coherent after each shock. Initially, I needed my heart shocked twice a day. Later, my doctors shared with me that I had gone into cardiopulmonary arrest, commonly called coding, over 25 times, and each time, my heart needed to be shocked to prevent sudden cardiac arrest.

Not surprisingly, my heart got weaker after each electric shock treatment. Years ago, this kind of cardiogenic shock would have been fatal but today, fifty percent of the people who experience heart shock survive with prompt treatment. One of the many things I did not know at the time was that I had a fifty percent chance of survival each time my heart was shocked. I learned that there is a clear connection between the heart's ability to recover and the amount of time before treatment; the longer the delay, the less heart muscle is maintained. We have all watched the medical dramas on television and movies where the doctors tell everyone to clear, so they can shock a person's heart. Well, I am here to let you know that in real life, it's not like those dramas. I felt like I was repeatedly kicked in the chest by a horse.

The doctors determined that the balloon pump wasn't working and I was taken back to the operating room for yet another procedure. My level of concern was rapidly increasing as I was not sure what's going on and why. However, I was also experiencing a bit of disbelief and hadn't had the opportunity to deal with this sudden illness. As with most things, I turned to humor as a defense mechanism and hide my insecurity with constant chatter. I was scared, but only those who knew me the best would know that I was just trying to deflect my fear by trying to be witty. I was hiding fear of dying behind a façade of humor and confidence. The surgeons removed the balloon pump from my left leg and then installed an Impella Heart Pump in my right leg. This new pump is stronger than the initial device, and with my declining heart function, it was determined that this was now needed to keep me alive. This pump was intended to be a short-term solution for a few hours; however, in some patients, an impella has been used to keep a patient alive for days, not months. Those around me knew that if I did not receive a new heart by the time the heart pump failed, I would more than likely pass away. The length of time the impella would work was not shared with me to protect me from knowing the number of days it would take before my heart finally fails. They knew that the added level of stress and despair would be too much for me.

Later that day, it was confirmed that I was suffering from acute heart failure due to Giant Cell Myocarditis (GCM). GCM is a rare, rapidly progressive viral infection where your body's immune system attacks your heart. To underscore the seriousness of this disease, I learned that GCM is often fatal and not discovered until an autopsy is performed. In the middle of all of this, I was intrigued and curious to learn about GCM and all the procedures being performed. I rapidly and frequently asked the residents, nurses, and anyone who would listen about the various procedures, equipment, and terms that were being used. Some of the team members look at me as if I was crazy, as if to say, 'does he not understand what is going on?' Others were more than happy to sit with me and explain in detail all that was happening as if "finally someone else is interested in this nerd stuff I love!"

"Let us not become weary in doing good, for at the proper time we will reap a harvest if we do not give up."

- Galatians 6:9 (NIV)

While the doctors were doing everything they could to keep me alive, my family was working with the transplant team to secure a place on the United Network for Organ Sharing (UNOS) national transplant waiting list. The number of steps, the quantity of information and interviews one goes through to even be considered for a transplant cannot be minimized. In 2018, only 3,133 of the more than 31,000 people that needed a heart transplant in the United States received one. Unfortunately, over 6,000 of the individuals on the transplant list pass away each day while waiting for an organ transplant (https://unos.org/).

Waiting times for transplants vary. The uniqueness of my condition and the outcome of the path I was on was of great interest to everyone at the hospital. Not everyone who needs a transplant will get one. This is because of the shortage of all organ types that are suitable for donation, only slightly more than fifty percent of the people on the waiting list will receive an organ within five years. To further place this in context, according to Goldstein, Thomas, Zaroff, Nguyen, Menza, & Khush (2016), patients on the waitlist with status 1A, 1, and 2 have median waiting times of 27, 71, and 252 days respectively. I was placed in status 1A on the waitlist on July 19, 2019. The transplant coordinator noted that I was the first patient in her experience to go straight to 1A status upon arrival. One of the most vivid memories of my time in the hospital was on July 23rd, when the director of the heart transplant program, Dr. J.

David Ortega, came to visit me in the ICU and told me that he was ninety-nine percent certain a heart was identified for me. The time between being placed on the transplant list and identification of a heart was also unheard of, if not incredibly rare. Remember, the national average time in 1A status to the identification of a heart is twenty-seven days; a heart was identified for me in only four.

A 2012 National Survey of Organ Donation Attitudes and Behaviors noted that only thirty-nine percent of African Americans were likely to check the box on their driver's license to allow their vital organs to be removed and transplanted after they die, while sixty-four percent of whites were likely to donate organs upon their death.

According to a September 18, 2018, article in US News, while black patients account for more than a quarter of those waiting for a kidney or a heart, members of the African American race make up less than fifteen percent of organ donor pools. According to the 2010 U.S. Census, Georgia had a population of 9,687,653. In terms of race, the population was: 59.7% White American (55.9% Non-Hispanic White, 3.8% White Hispanic), 30.5% Black or African American).

Generations of mistrust of the medical field is a major factor for the low organ donation rates among African Americans. There are a vast number of examples, but I will only highlight three. In the 1800s, Dr. James Sims used enslaved African women as subjects for women's reproductive system experiments. Early accounts of Dr. Sim's work tell of barbaric practices where he perfected a technique to repair complications within women's reproductive tracts by repeatedly conducting painful experimental surgeries on enslaved black women without using anesthesia. The outcomes of these practices led to advances in women's health and to Dr. Sims being considered the father of modern gynecology (Ojanuga, 1993). In 1932, the Alabama Department of Public Health began a study to determine the natural course of untreated Syphilis in the Male Negro. Despite the revelation that penicillin was available and would help, the men infected were not offered this treatment. After a large number of men died, the experiment was discontinued in 1972, after the public became aware of this tragedy (Fairchild & Bayer, 1999). In the 1950s, scientists at Johns Hopkins Hospital created the first immortal human cell line with a tissue sample taken from a young black woman with cervical cancer. The piece of her tumor was taken without her consent. These immortal human cells became essential to developing the polio vaccine and were later used for advances in cloning, gene mapping, and in vitro fertilization. It wasn't until the 1970s that the world became aware that these advances in medicine were a result of this black woman, who was not given credit or compensation for the work performed with her cells (Lucey, Nelson-Rees, & Hutchins, 2009).

The United States has a history of racial bias, including the unequal treatment of African Americans by physicians and hospitals. I would argue that African American's attitudes toward organ donation will begin to change as a result of both education around the needs and benefits to our community related to organ donation, coupled with an increasing number of positive experiences and outcomes when dealing with the medical community. Another barrier to African American's organ donation is a desire to target the donation. When I talked to people during the writing of this book, I repeatedly heard from African Americans that they don't agree to organ donation simply because they cannot be assured that their organ(s) will be donated to another African American. Recognizing the need for increased organ donation at death, the American Medical Association (AMA) approved policies in 2017 to create educational programs designed to address myths and concerns in communities that historically have low donation rates.

6.

"The Lord sustains them on their sickbed and restores them from their bed of illness."

- Psalm 41:3 (NIV)

My surgical team was the best I could have hoped for. They performed rounds at 7:00 a.m. each morning. The lead surgeon, Dr. Ortega, would stop by early to see how I did overnight and update his directions to the team, which included my medicine or meal restrictions. Later in the morning, a larger group of physicians and medical students would come by to discuss each case; they became known as the TMZ crew (The Crew). The TMZ Crew earned that nickname because of the way they usually formed a circle and discussed each case; their approach was reminiscent lar entertainment television show. My wife was

ᵤᵢn *The Crew* of doctors with various specialties to

hear what was going on in great detail. As the days went by and my condition worsened, *The Crew* began discussing options for prolonging my life. A blood transfusion was one option but not the preferred approach. The challenge with a transfusion is that when a transplant is performed, there would be less blood in the body system, which would increase the likelihood of rejection. During this entire time, I was only vaguely aware of what was going on, partially because I was being shielded from things that might have created additional anxiety due to the fact that I was in and out of consciousness. I would waver between being happy and sad as I was just trying to hold on to life.

My daughters would come in the room and I would simply look at them and smile, then I would cry. I was concerned that I was going to miss watching them graduate from school, would not be there to walk them down the aisle on their wedding days, or miss seeing my eventual grandchildren. My parents passed away before my daughters were born and I feared history was repeating itself. On a normal day, we often take these things for granted, but when you feel as if your days are numbered, your feelings became more in tune with the finality of death and every life event becomes more important.

While all of the medical procedures were taking place, additional meetings were taking place between my family and various members of the team as a part of the heart transplant evaluation process. The assessment process is a lengthy and detailed process that qualifies people for a new organ. The heart transplant coordinators facilitated meetings with financial counselors, physical therapists, and physiologists. The hospital requested for my medical records, dental records, and several others. Questions asked ranged from our financial capacity, family stability, support structure, mental stability, work history, and my childhood environment, to name a few. My dentist and primary care physician moved heaven and earth to ensure that my medical history was submitted by 10:00 a.m. on the 19th of July. The extensive interview process, coupled with my health status, was used to determine if I would be a candidate for the transplant list and at what level. There are multiple levels to the transplant list:

- Status 1A or urgent need requiring intensive care hospitalization, life-support measures, certain cardiac supporting intravenous medications or mechanical-assist device(s).

- Status 1B: The patient is dependent on intravenous medications or a mechanical-assist device – in the hospital or at home.
- Status 2: Stable on oral medications and able to wait at home and
- Status 7 or the inactive list: Inactive due to a change in condition – patients do not lose time they have already accrued.

To keep my mind of all that was happening and the range of outcomes, I found myself praying, listening to music, and doing anything I could think of to pass the time. Now, I was on the other side and have to be mindful of caring for my new heart, but there were many significant challenges for patients on the waitlist to receive a new life-saving organ. Doctors Aslam & Mehra also expressed concerns regarding how COVID-19 will affect organ donation. Others argue that assessing the organ donor's health prior to receiving an organ has become increasingly difficult (coronavirus.gov). I watched how the donation process could be a complicated and long process for some in the pre-COVID-19 environment. Doctors were worried that they now have to consider whether the donor had been exposed or infected with the coronavirus and the implications for the person in need of it and potentially receiving the donated organ.

In addition, the often-reported stress placed on the medical community, the availability of beds, equipment, and other resources also adds to the risk for recipients waiting on this life-saving measure. While COVID-19 has changed life as we knew it, the already complicated process to care for those with transplanted organs and those waiting on new organs has been intensified.

Finally, be strong in the Lord and in his mighty power. Put on the full armor of God, so that you can take your stand against the devil's schemes. For our struggle is not against flesh and blood, but against the rulers, against the authorities, against the powers of this dark world and against the spiritual forces of evil in the heavenly realms.

Therefore put on the full armor of God, so that when the day of evil comes, you may be able to stand your ground, and after you have done everything, to stand. Stand firm then, with the belt of truth buckled around your waist, with the breastplate of righteousness in place, and with your feet fitted with the readiness that comes from the gospel of peace.

Dr. Arthur D. Vaughn

In addition to all this, take up the shield of faith, with which you can extinguish all the flaming arrows of the evil one. Take the helmet of salvation and the sword of the Spirit, which is the word of God.

- Ephesians 6:10-17 (NIV)

The Senior Pastor and Executive Pastor from our church — whom we also consider friends — came to visit with me on multiple occasions. We would chat and they prayed with me. They recommended a Bible app that I downloaded, so I could listen to scripture when I did not have the strength to sit up and read. The pastoral staff from the hospital would also stop by and chat with the transplant team and me. I was surrounded by believers and felt protected by the armor of God. I learned a new level of faith and knew that if I lived or died, I would surely be at peace. However, as I told the coordinators, I was not ready to go just yet.

The transplant coordinators played a major role in the pre-surgery process and continue to be vital in my recovery. These wonderful ladies were there from the start, providing education to my family and working closely to ensure that we made it through what seemed to be a complex series of paperwork that allowed me to receive a donor's heart. I also learned that the team also acted to ease the burden on the donors' family's and educate them — who I believe had to be going through the worst time of their lives as well. While managing all of these moving parts, the team of guardian angels had to be in constant communication with the surgeons, doctors, nurses, and other administrators during the pre-transplant process. After the surgery, my family told me about all of the work the coordinators had done, as I was too ill prior to the surgery to fully contribute to the process. However, after I regained consciousness — and ever since — I have been able to work directly with them regarding my care and recuperation.

During moments when I felt pain, experienced setbacks, had questions about my medications, or any number of other issues, they always supported me and I began to feel like they are a part of my extended family. Frankly, there were a couple of times when I was scared, in pain, or sleep-deprived when my words were not kind and did not reflect the appreciation I have for these remarkable people that were there all through my tough moments. Despite my low points, these ladies have shown nothing but professionalism, care, and compassion.

7.

"My flesh and my heart may fail, but God is the strength of my heart and my portion forever."

- Psalm 73:26 (NIV)

I t was determined that I would be placed on the list in 1A status, meaning that the next compatible heart within 500 nautical miles would be mine. Each day after being placed on the transplant list, I prayed for another day and for a heart to become available. Later, this prayer would haunt me as I began to process that someone else had to die that I may live. The sacrifice another family had to experience still torments me to this day.

Four days after being placed on the transplant list, my surgeon informed me that the hospital was ninety-nine percent certain they had a heart that matched my needs. Uncharacteristically, I began to slap Dr. Ortega on his chest and say, "Thank you, thank you, and thank you!" Those around were a bit in awe as no one had ever seen this physician, who is held in such high esteem, treated in such a common manner by a patient. The doctors told me that my new heart wasn't perfect since the donor was a weed smoker. I told the doctors that I smoked a few cigars, so we would call it even.

My girls came to the hospital and for the first time, my true condition was shared with them. Before this, the girls knew I was sick and in the hospital, but they did not know that I was more likely to die than to live. Later that evening, a portion of the medical team came to my room to begin prepping me for surgery. I was excited; it's going to happen — I am going to get a new heart. For the last twenty-four hours, I wasn't able to focus on the ninety-nine percent likelihood that I was getting a heart. I wasn't sure why, but my mind was in a glass-half-empty mode. I was afraid of what was going to happen if that one percent chance of not getting a heart became a reality.

The team rolled me from my room to the operating room with my family in tow. As I understand it, the Care and Comfort Pastor from our church joined my family as they waited patiently for me to be operated on. She had spent many days and nights with me at the hospital prior to my surgery and has visited a number of times afterward. One last wave, I went left to the operating room and they went right to the waiting room. Once in the operating room, you go into the "hurry up and wait" mode. They clean you up and begin connecting you to the various machines and lines they will need to help get you through this process.

On the fifth day after being placed on the transplant list, I spent hours lying flat on my back on the cold and hard surgical table while the team verified the usefulness of the heart. The anesthesiologist then placed a mask over my face and asked me to count backward from ten. I don't think I counted to seven before I became unconscious! The machines had kept me alive for two weeks and on July 24, 2019, I had a new heart!

8.

"Peace I leave with you; my peace I give you. I do not give to you as the world gives. Do not let your hearts be troubled and do not be afraid."

- John 14:27 (NIV)

The next thing I remember was waking up in the ICU on a ventilator with a breathing tube and other tubes sticking out of my chest, my hands tied down, and the inability to communicate. One of the greatest fears one can have is having their breath taken away. I imagined that this is what it must feel like to drown. I have heard stories about how people wake up alarmed due to the lack of control of their arms because they are tied down to the bed. I was slowly waking up and becoming aware of where I was. At the time, I was not thinking about why the tube was there and how it helped me breathe during the surgery. My mind began to race and fight; I wanted to pull away and regain control. I was becoming increasingly agitated when I heard a whisper in my ear — a voice that has been a guiding force in my life for over twenty years — my wife. Her voice brought a sense of stillness over me and I began to close my eyes and relax. I could not see her clearly, but I believe that she leaned over to my ear and simply said, "Relax. . . and if you relax for just a little while, the doctors will be able to remove the breathing tube." I followed her voice and gave in to the experience, allowed my mind to become extremely peaceful, and the tubes were removed.

As I continued to regain consciousness, some disturbing questions raced through my mind: Where did this heart come from? Why did someone else's child have to die so I could live? I became sober and didn't want to see anyone the morning I woke up. I wasn't ready to see my kids, my siblings, friends, or anyone else the morning after surgery. Not everyone understood this feeling that overwhelmed me; I am not sure I understood it then and I am still not sure I do. This was confusing to my family members who had traveled to be with me during my time of need, but it was what I needed at the moment. They wrapped me in a cocoon of love that allowed me to get from diagnoses to transplant, but my mind was in distress, as I was trying to process what had happened. I had been so weak in body and spirit prior to the surgery that I hadn't processed any of what was going on. I remembered being admitted to the hospital, and I will never forget the first time I was coded and shocked into a normal rhythm. But most of what occurred from the time I was admitted to the hospital and up until the surgery remained unclear to me. My mind was telling me that I died multiple times. Each electric shock to my heart felt like a death and rebirth. While I laid in bed preceding the surgery, my mind was in a constant cycle of confusion.

The first night after my transplant, I did not sleep at all. I hadn't reconciled the fact that my failed heart had been replaced with a perfectly healthy heart. I could not accept that I was alive because someone else had died. I felt that if I allowed myself to go to sleep, my heart would fail and I would die in my sleep. I watched television, stared at the walls, the ceilings, and just gazed into space. As I laid in the bed barely conscious, all sorts of images and ideas ran through my head. I was afraid that if I didn't stay awake, I wouldn't wake up. I believed I had conversations with others, saying I was gone and wishing them well. I believed I had met with my daughters and said, "Goodbye. . . take care of your mother." I believed I had died. This was the first of several instances that I needed help with the state of grief I was experiencing. I wasn't ready to see anyone and receive any cover of healing love. I knew that I had one of the most amazing support systems anyone could ask for, but I wasn't ready to face them this time.

This feeling stayed with me for months after surgery and still haunts me to this day. The anxiety, lack of sleep, and overall sense of guilt surfaced all at once the next morning. That morning, I was struggling emotionally and it was evident. Unconsciously, I knew I was different, the pain from my failed heart was no longer there because the last thing I could remember was a sense of weakness and fragility with a feeling that I was likely to die. Then a rush of regret and emotion flowed over me. I do not recall what set everything off, but the doctor asked me if I was all right and needed anything. I remember simply just losing it, franticly crying and screaming uncontrollably saying, "I need help, I need help! I need help!" At that moment, my mental health journey began.

9.

"For it is by grace you have been saved, through faith—and this is not from yourselves, it is the gift of God—not by works, so that no one can boast."

- Ephesians 2:8-9 (NIV)

Two things became strikingly clear to me that morning—physical health cannot be detached from one's mental health. When we are not mentally strong, it is difficult to heal physically. I didn't realize that I was experiencing a psychotic episode until much later. I was struggling to process what had happened. I was scared, especially as I had so many unfamiliar people around me. My response was not physical, but an emotional reaction that consumed me like a waterfall. The feeling of dying and being reborn was like a rush that I wasn't prepared to handle.

I tried to put everything that transpired over the last ten to fourteen days in context. When you think of it, my whirlwind from sickness to a healthy physical state all occurred over a period of time, which is equivalent to some people's family vacation. I was not afforded the time to process what was happening, and when I was at my lowest point, I wasn't conscious enough to always know what was going on. I went from being a relatively healthy fifty-year-old man to being on the brink of death and then brought back to life. However, in all of these, I never want anyone to feel sorry for me. I am alive by God's grace with an opportunity to continue to live. It's a feeling, a moment that lives so vividly in my mind for eternity. For the second time, I heard the whisper in my ear. Octavia placed her hands on both sides of my face, leaned over, and said, "Look at me! You need to listen to me! The first thing you are going to do is stop this and calm down. You are going to do it now! You are disturbing everyone on the floor." On cue, I went silent. She then said, "I am going to tell you the facts, what happened, and what didn't happen." She went on to share with me the events of the last week and conversations I had with our daughters and others. She shared with me what was real, what

I imagined, and brought me back to the truth. For me, this was a form of therapy — a safe harbor during an abundance of unchecked emotion.

My family and various close friends were now able to visit me. Friends from near and far stepped up without being asked to support my family through prayer, monetary gifts, and good works. My early recovery was unconventional, to say the least. A couple of days after having the breathing tube removed, I was able to move to the chair in the ICU. I ended up staying in that chair for days as I refused to return to the hospital bed. The experience of the last few weeks in that hospital bed represented a place of pain, helplessness, loss of control, and fear.

Heart transplants are not a cure for a disease. They are a trade-off from one medical problem that a person can no longer live with for another that can be medically managed. After my various procedures and surgeries, there were instances when I questioned: "Why me? What did I do to deserve this new heart?" This was the beginning of my journey to understanding God's Favor. Over the next several months, my mind was filled with thoughts and ideas I never had to deal with, such as the meaning of life after my death. Understanding how quickly the condition took hold of my body, how close to death I was, and how blessed I was to receive a second chance at life were all emotional struggles I had to work through over time and often with assistance from multiple mental health professionals. The psychological complexities of the medicines I was administered also contributed to the altered mental state I suffered from time to time. My changing family dynamics also complicated my recovery.

For I was hungry and you gave me nothing to eat, I was thirsty and you gave me nothing to drink, I was a stranger and you did not invite me in, I needed clothes and you did not clothe me, I was sick and in prison and you did not look after me.' "They also will answer, 'Lord, when did we see you hungry or thirsty or a stranger or needing clothes or sick or in prison, and did not help you?' "He will reply, 'Truly I tell you, whatever you did not do for one of the least of these, you did not do for me."

- Matthew 25:42-45 (NIV)

The physicians, nurses, and medical staff at the hospital are top-notch, and I couldn't have been cared for at a better place.

The nurses are lifesavers, a highly trained set of superheroes in navy blue that deal with people at their lowest point in life. Every patient comes into the hospital at different levels of illness, and the hospital providers employ their special set of skills to get each of us back to our optimal health. I asked one Cardiovascular Intensive Care Nurse (ICU) nurse why he opted to be in this field. In response, he said, "We deal with issues related to patient care. In the ICU, people are at their worse and our job is to help them get better. When they get to the recovery floor (The Floor), patients are better and the nurses on the floor work with people to prepare them for their transition home."

My journey has been filled with unmerited favor, God's grace, and blessings. However, it hasn't been void of humbling experiences. While in the ICU, I was so weak that I had to regularly ask the nursing staff to sit me on the toilet and clean me up afterward. For any independent person, this experience would be humbling, but I saw myself as superhuman — with no obstacle beyond my ability to conquer. For the most part, the hospital nursing staff handled this with professionalism and kindness each time they tended to me. They ensured I was clean and comfortable with the exception of a couple of experiences.

One afternoon I laid in the bed, unable to move much and

needed help to be positioned in a way that would make me feel comfortable. This may seem minor, but after the previous fourteen-day ordeal, ten hours of surgery, and generally not knowing what was going on around me, the simple comforts were incredibly important. As a result of the physical trauma and the various medications in my system, I was in a heightened emotional state, to say the least. I was experiencing a great deal of anxiety while lying in a broken bed, and from my perspective, no one was willing to help. After I asked the nurse responsible for my care for help, a second nurse entered the room. Now, instead of assisting me, they engaged in a conversation about the manufacturing and defects in my broken hospital bed. I felt disregarded and distressed as I laid soiled in the bed while the nurse ignored me and attended to other duties. I snapped! I told them both my care should be first and that I didn't give a damn about the history of the *fucking* bed. Until someone showed care for me, the history of the bed and the other trivial things they were discussing did not matter to me. After a while, the content and volume of my comments drew others to the room; the lead nurse was empathetic to my concerns and was very apologetic. After I had displayed my rage, a much larger team of nurses cleaned me up, adjusted me in the bed, and ensured I was comfortable. But it was too late. I was in the midst of another emotional break.

Later that week, my second collision with the nursing staff occurred. My arm and leg muscles, having gone through a certain level of deterioration from a lack of use, meant that I was unable to stand on my own. This was yet another night I had to be helped to the portable toilet. After having a bowel movement, I was unable to properly clean myself. I was left sitting on this rigid, plastic seat for what in my mind was thirty minutes while the nurse focused on completing charts and ignored my requests to clean me up. The nurse's rationale was she did not think I was finished despite my statements to the contrary. I lost my cool again. My perception was that I was being treated less than human. I was immobile, unclean, and ashamed.

Again, a larger team of nurses came to my room and some attempted to rationalize the initial nurse's behavior. I made it clear that my feelings should not be marginalized and that no one should attempt to explain away what I was feeling. My feelings were real to me. How we are made to feel is always valid. While the nurse's actions were not intentionally designed to make me feel less than human, they were all real to me at that point. It is a daunting task to manage the rush of emotions and everything that is going on around you while accepting the life-changing trauma that was experienced. My ability to shave, shower, and clean myself were things I took for granted and I was looking forward to being able to do them again.

I know I am not the first to go through all of this, but until you do, I strongly believe most of us do not have an appreciation for those who have such a life-altering incident. I think it's important for me to end this by noting that these were exceptions. Overall, the nursing staff cared for me at a level beyond my expectations; their compassion and empathy were only exceeded by their professionalism and skill. I have photos and fond memories of several of the nursing staff that cared for me deeply and can't thank them enough for nurturing me back to health.

I couldn't help but think of my experience through the lens of those who haven't had the same exposure and experience I have had, some who how don't even know that the treatment I received isn't acceptable. I began to verbally advocate for those who struggle to advocate for themselves. These few experiences remind me that those of us who understand the plight of the less fortunate, those of us with means, those of us with resources, and those who have a platform must continue to advocate for equity in care. We have to use our voices to support others who are blessed in different ways, and whom we can relieve from some of their burdens.

10.

"But he said to me, "My grace is sufficient for you, for my power is made perfect in weakness." Therefore I will boast all the more gladly about my weaknesses, so that Christ's power may rest on me."

- 2 Corinthians 12:9

Today, I moved from the cardiovascular intensive care unit (ICU) to the Cardiac Care Unit (CCU), also referred to as "The Floor." Being moved to *The Floor* means I was now officially a short-timer in the hospital. More importantly, this meant that all of the annoying and uncomfortable tubes and wires would be removed — signifying that my new heart is stable and working. The doctors were now comfortable that I was not experiencing rejection and my heart no longer needed to be shocked. Normally, when my surgeon completes doing God's work by saving another life in the operating room, it is expected of him to submit the order to remove my last remaining tubes. The optics related to the chest tubes and the bloody fluid being pumped from my body was intimidating. This was a huge milestone and my family and I were overjoyed. One of the other surgeons on the team, Dr. Miller, stopped by that morning and placed the last month of activity in a way that I truly appreciated: "Three weeks ago you were fine and enjoying life. Then you were clinging to life, and five days ago, you got a transplant and a new life." To some, that may seem very a matter of fact. To me, Dr. Miller's words reaffirmed the power of God. I want to research all the data about what caused my heart to fail — the mortality rate and the treatment — but there is never enough time or I find myself too tired.

It wasn't until I was moved out of the ICU that I slept through the night and in the bed. My first night on *The Floor*, I slept in the chair as I had done almost every night since surgery. The hospital bed represented illness and death to me; it was something that made me fearful and anxious. My second night on *The Floor* was the first time I wanted to sleep in the hospital bed. This was the first time since the surgery that the bed became a source of comfort and rest. I slept for six hours until the usual 4:30 a.m. blood draw by the nursing staff. The nursing staff would come back at 6:00 a.m. to give me some medicine and check my vital signs before the shift changed at 7:00 a.m. I learned quickly that if I wanted to get any sleep, I needed to go bed between 9:30 p.m. or 10:00 p.m. They were on a schedule, and it wasn't going to be disrupted by my desire to sleep. After a period when I could not sleep at all, I slept five to six hours per day and found myself able to rest and write. . . and began getting ready for physical and mental therapy. All of the connections that had been inserted or attached to my body were removed except the heart monitors. The images and feelings related to being helpless, weak, and without control remained vivid in my mind. The tubes had also been reminders that I am still healing mentally. I was writing four months after being discharged from the hospital, but the feelings of anguish from being connected to the machines were still very real in my mind.

Soon after being moved to *The Floor,* my next major milestone was scheduled with the cardiologist performing a heart biopsy. The completion of the biopsy is another procedure that signifies that my discharge date was rapidly approaching. This procedure was one that was eventually be performed on me so many times it became routine. The surgeon used a local anesthetic to deaden an area between the lower portion of my neck and chest plate. Using a needle, the physician ran a probe from the incision — where microscopic tissue samples of my heart were taken and tested for infection and rejection. Each time a piece of my heart was taken, I felt as if I could feel it. I felt as if I had a minor heart fluctuation and that part of me would never be the same.

"You are standing here in order to enter into a covenant with the Lord your God, a covenant the Lord is making with you this day and sealing with an oath."

- Deuteronomy 29:12 (NIV)

In the days after transitioning to *The Floor*, inpatient physical therapy was set to begin. Over the past eighteen days, I had been bedridden and I gradually began was walking across the floor. It is truly humbling when you realize how weak your muscles become in such a short period of time. I had to work hard to perform simple tasks I previously took for granted, like standing on my own, walking across the room, and running. In the early days on *The Floor*, standing was a major task. The team got me out of bed and moving in this fancy walker. It was emotionally overpowering at first, but after moving, it felt great. My balance returned quickly, and with the support of the machine, I was able to walk a short distance. It would be months before my legs were strong enough to stand for a period of time, and even longer before I could run. During the initial rehabilitation period, my greatest accomplishments turned out to be my biggest curse. I exceeded every goal and blew away every milestone the therapist would set. I was even exceeding my own expectations. The premature successes led to my inability to have the appropriate appreciation for all I had gone through, which led me not to respect the process it will take for me to truly recover.

The next day was incredibly long. There was a steady and overlapping group of people visiting my room. Technicians came by to draw blood for lab work, physical and occupational therapists, social workers, transplant specialists, pharmacists, and x-ray technicians all stopped by before I saw the team of cardiologists for the day. It's now nine days after surgery, and I was ready to be discharged from the hospital. Up to this point, everything had been managed by others who understood my wishes. To no surprise, there were no missteps and things were handled in the manner I would have wanted if I had completed the steps myself.

The bureaucracy that we had to work through before being discharged could intimidate anyone. The sheer volume and complexity of the paperwork required to ensure the medical bills were paid and my disability benefits could be paid out. At times, I felt like the volume of paperwork was designed to deter and disqualify beneficiaries instead of simplifying coverage for the insured. I felt that despite being covered by one of the largest insurers in the world, I began to think the fictitious and fraudulent company "Great Benefit" of the J.J. Abrams film *The Rainmaker* had insured me. I learned many lessons during my illness, and one critically important one thing I found was that we should always document and make known our desires should we become ill. I believe we should write down who is to make medical decisions for us when we cannot make our wishes known regarding cremation or burial and have a will that dictates how any assets we have are to be distributed. I did not have all of this in order as I never saw this illness coming; we never do. I was in the process of ensuring that this was done going forward so that my family is provided for when my time does come.

"I will praise you, Lord, with all my heart; before the "gods" I will sing your praise."

- Psalm 138:1 (NIV)

It was discharge day and I was super excited! It was a quiet day and with the use of a high tech walking support machine, I walked three laps around the floor just to keep myself busy — I was ready to go home and be around my familiar surroundings, as I haven't felt the sun on my face or breathed the outside air in a month. When the nursing staff rolled me outside in the wheelchair, I just wanted to sit and be in the moment. I sat still, closed my eyes, and let the warmth of Georgia's summer sun hit my face. I was in heaven after a month of hell.

11.

The ride home was quiet and I did some sightseeing while taking in the tree-lined streets in the North Druid Hills section of Atlanta. When I arrived, I wanted my bare feet to touch our freshly cut grass. I wanted to see my home, my place of peace, and my castle for the past twenty years. It's amazing how you don't appreciate these simple things until they are taken from you. This is a consistent theme in our lives, but it doesn't seem to become real until it happens. I remember arriving home and watching all the activity going on around with a sense of excitement.

The support we received did not end when I was discharged from the hospital. When I arrived home after being hospitalized for twenty-five days, there was a young man — who my eldest daughter has known since birth — waiting to help me up the stairs and in the house. Climbing those three stairs was incredibly tasking and it left me tired and breathing heavily. The aftermath of simply getting from the car to the front door should have let me know that things would not return to "normal" quickly. The number of get-well cards, meals delivered to our home, and calls to check on our family was really awesome.

I slept like a rock on my first night at home post-surgery. Interestingly enough, my sleep pattern mirrored the last few days in the hospital, but the sleep was sounder. I woke up around 4:25 a.m. for just a few moments and then knocked out until 7:45 a.m. During this time, I noticed the rhythm and beat of my new heart. I quietly listened to my heart beating as I moved around the house. It was something I do not believe I paid attention to in the past, but now I was aware of every beat. I was home and eager because I would be taking a shower and shave. The simplest of things were pleasures I got excited about. Things I took for granted became special occasions.

Not only was it my first day back home, it was also my Octavia's first day back at home. She spent every night at the hospital with me, participated in every meeting and procedure to the extent to which she could. We were adjusting together.

Later that day, I was afforded the opportunity to sit outside for a bit. The warmth of the sun and southern air was refreshing. I then attempted a short walk around the property. My early attempts to walk were constant reminders that all of this was still new and the challenge was real — this is the beginning of a long journey. My legs remained weak from the muscle atrophy I experienced from being bedridden. I could only imagine the physical toll those who are restricted to bed for periods of months and rehabilitation program must have endured to get back to being themselves. During my recovery, my weight dropped to a low of 209 lbs. down from 262 lbs I weighed when I entered the hospital. My legs lacked muscle, yet I began to move slowly and work hard to get my muscles strong, nursing the goal of running in my ninth Atlanta Peachtree Road Race a year to the month after my surgery.

I had to learn to respect the recovery process and take my time healing. While I could not exercise my body the way I may have wanted to, I thought my mind was still sharp and ready to go. I was wrong. After talking with the physicians, I learned some never returned to their old form. The damage sustained became too much for some and they were never the same.

Dr. Arthur D. Vaughn

"Let the wise listen and add to their learning, and let the discerning get guidance—"

- Proverbs 1:5 (NIV)

The large quantities of steroids I was given were making me feel loopy and incoherent. The medical team warned me that my new medications might also cause mental challenges. I was emotionally struggling to adjust to the steroids I was taking to prevent my immune system from attacking my heart. When I initially walked out of the hospital, I was feeling strong and determined to get back to my old life. I was ready to resume my meeting and activity schedule, so I began scheduling meetings and attending events. I felt like I could take one meeting per week at home and continue to be who I was prior to becoming ill. But instead of the high energy person I was, my energy level was low and my pain grew even worse. I was not listening to my body or those around me. I needed to learn for myself that rest and releasing myself from prior obligations was needed to facilitate my healing.

The agony I was in was eased when my great uncle stopped by with my mother-in-law the next day. I really enjoy spending time with and chatting with my elders; I recognized more than ever that senior members of our family wouldn't always be here. Following my first month out of the hospital, I felt really great. I would go out to the park and walk a brisk mile without my legs being wobbly when I finished. There would be times during my walk when I would want to stop, but I would tell myself not to quit.

You were taught, with regard to your former way of life, to put off your old self, which is being corrupted by its deceitful desires; to be made new in the attitude of your minds; and to put on the new self, created to be like God in true righteousness and holiness.

- Ephesians 4:22-24 (NIV)

It's crazy. When I first came home from the hospital, I wanted nothing more than to have the warmth of the sun hit my face. A month later, this summer humidity and the consistent ninety plus degree weather made it difficult to breathe whenever I went outside, though I preferred it to staying back in the house, which felt like I was in captivity. During the times my breathing was labored, I used a breathing machine to help me get through the day. That breathing machine was a godsend during this time of heavy air and record-setting heat.

It's common for transplant patients to call this regular appointment "Hospital Day." During my first follow-up appointment post-transplant, the healthcare providers did the normal blood work and heart biopsy. When I went in for a heart biopsy, the team numbed an area at the bottom of my neck and above my collarbone. They inserted a probe in this space and navigate down to my heart. There were times when they checked the pressure around my heart and other times when they took microscopic pieces of the heart to examine and ascertain if my body was rejecting my new heart. It was interesting that all of these procedures became a routine for me, but when I describe them to friends, they are all amazed by the progress I made thus far. The restrictions, the medication regime, the blood tests, and the doctor's appointments were now just a normal way of life.

The wait time between the procedure and the results was always tense. Rejection meant I needed to undergo additional treatments to ensure my body accepts the new heart. When I think of rejection, I think of the three weeks in July, where I sat and wondered if I would live or die. The mental anxiety and stress of not knowing what was going to happen created a sense of helplessness, as I could control the outcome. During this time, I was led to explore my core beliefs and to let go and let God direct my healing. A day or so later, we found out the results of this biopsy and it showed zero rejection. At this point, my body adjusted to my initial period of rejection and began accepting the new heart without any complications.

I did not know what was going on, as I did not know what I was supposed to feel like after surgery. Previously, I could sense when my body wasn't functioning like "normal." This new normal was not defined yet, so I did not know what feeling weird felt like. Right now, everything felt weird. A number of the drugs I was taking were designed to weaken my immune system, while the others are intended to compensate for the side effects of the anti-rejection medicine.

My initial diagnoses, the fact I lived, and the post-operation treatment of my giant cell were clearly of interest as I had the privilege of working with a team of cardiac transplant physicians, a team of infectious disease physicians, and a team of neuroscience physicians throughout my recovery. During hospital day, the providers ran blood tests and did heart biopsies to check for rejection. The hospital day was usually on

Thursdays, and this point, they ran my normal test and I figured I would be in and out. That wouldn't be the case today.

After the normal procedures were run, one of the doctors came in and shared that antibodies are building up for the second week in a row, and if this week's blood test doesn't show a decline, I will need to be admitted for six days for aggressive treatment. I assumed that this was just another hurdle, as I felt stronger than I had since the surgery was performed. Similar to my initial diagnoses, my body was preparing to attack this new heart. I would be lying if I say I wasn't concerned about all of these changes. Rejection can have many consequences, ranging from a temporary illness to death. I began thinking of all that happened in July. The quickness with which I became ill, the weakness, the in and out of consciousness, and the inability to function or care for myself are fresh in my mind. My mental state went from a place of strength to one that was incredibly delicate. However, the doctors were concerned but not worried. While I was mentally comprised, I am physically ready for this challenge, and when we got home, I began to prepare for a one-week stay in the hospital and told myself, *let God's will be done!*

They increased the dosages of the anti-rejection medicines, which in turn suppressed my immune system and caused a weight gain. No one said recovery would be easy — and in addition to the biopsy, lab work, and EKG, the doctors added a right-heart-pressure test to my regular routine. I was told that the blood work wasn't complete, but the biopsy results are in. I was also told that the tests show moderate to severe levels of rejection, which scared me. What I heard was: "You have rejection, and you are headed to another month like July." Every day in July was the worst day of my life and I expected it to be my last. My heart was failing more and more to the point machines that were keeping me alive. Rejection to me is equivalent to the beginning of failure, and the comfortable way it was shared showed an absence of understanding and empathy for what I was going through.

Thoughts of all of the procedures, the shocking of my heart, weakness, and death dominated my mind. I knew that if another month like rolled by, I won't be able to survive it, and if I can, it just won't be now. Six weeks ago, I was as close to death as I could have been, and I was told that my body was rejecting my new heart.

12.

019 was the tale of two years. During the first half, I was flying by the seat of my pants — hanging out, golf, cigars, parties, and living what some call the "good life." That good life came with being away from my family, neglecting my responsibilities at home, and not being the man I was supposed to be. In the 4th quarter of the year, everything had fallen apart. I was in a slow recovery from an unexpected heart transplant, multiple bouts with my body rejecting my new heart, and my home life had fallen apart. The feelings of despair and sorrow were gradually taking its toll on me.

As I sat in the parking lot of the local big box home improvement store, my mind immediately reflected on my last visit to this same store. It was early evening, maybe thirty minutes before closing time and I had stopped by to pick up some hardware — that a week later, I still hadn't installed. I stepped out of the car, and as I walked, I began feeling dizzy. I attempted to get back to the truck so that I could use it as a support. However, I didn't make it and found myself flat on my back on the cold concrete. I laid there for a few minutes until my blood pressure equalized and I was able to move. Then, I made it in to the store, quickly grabbed the hardware, and slowly made my way back to the truck. That wasn't the first or last dizzy spell I experienced. These issues of unbalanced blood pressure happened fairly regularly. I had to remember my blood vessels were reattached, but my nerve endings could not be attached during surgery. As a result of not having the nerves connected, it took a moment for my brain and heart to get in sync when I wanted to move. Until the two organs linked up, my body couldn't properly respond.

After treatment for rejection, I went from regularly walking two miles to struggling to walk across the room without the use of a cane. My hands had become shaky and I was losing focus intermittently. I was scheduled to return to work but delayed it to another month with the hope that some of the symptoms will further subside. In order to help facilitate my healing, I asked the doctors to sign me up for cardiac rehabilitation. One of the challenges with rehabilitation was that it was group-focused and not personalized, based on where each person is in their recovery. Throughout the process, I have been ahead of the curve, so I stopped attending cardiac rehabilitation. I began working out on my own by doing thirty minutes of cardio three times per week while drinking no less than two liters of water. While it may be unconventional for someone at this stage, my physicians approved my workout based on my condition. Even now, I find it difficult to focus and my hands are still shaking.

Post-transplant, I've had bouts with anger, depression, and anxiety. Unfortunately, I was also dealing with the decline of my 20-year marriage at the same time, which complicated my recovery from the physical and emotional trauma I experienced. However, with the help of a therapist, I began to address a number of issues associated with the grief I was experiencing. Through therapy, I began to understand the root causes of the issues I needed to work through and how I was expressing them in my daily life. My weekly therapy sessions with Dr. Parkins helped provide me with coping mechanisms that helped with emotional outbursts that randomly occurred without warning. However, over time, the sessions with a therapist were not enough and I began seeing a psychiatrist as well.

Dr. Arthur D. Vaughn

When you pass through the waters, I will be with you; and when you pass through the rivers, they will not sweep over you. When you walk through the fire, you will not be burned; the flames will not set you ablaze.

- Isaiah 43:2 (NIV)

It had been less than six months since my transplant and the biopsy results came in — I was experiencing rejection for the second time. I cried out of frustration after I heard the news and then sucked it up, which meant I would have to go back to the hospital for three days of treatment. I continued to have faith in God, and His guidance was made real in the doctors' and nurses' hands. Physically, I was weak, but I had to move through that. My biggest issue continued to be my mental state as I struggled daily with social distancing and emotional isolation. This is a serious condition that has affected me hugely and I am taking it seriously, but I have to deal with it my way and not the ways others think I should.

The anger I was feeling became obvious, and I needed to get away from my reality that evening, so I went to the movies for a nice two-hour reprieve. I am not being defeatist, but this is the second battle with rejection since being initially discharged from the hospital. I can't help but think that eventually, my immune system was going to win. My native heart was attacked and killed by my immune system. My system was clearly strong, and I wondered if the various medicines would be able to depress my system, and if the system is consistently weakened, are there other viruses such as COVID-19 out there that will end up killing me?

Later that day, the doctors became a bit indecisive as to whether or not I was in rejection and they were unclear about the course of treatment. The doctor's tentativeness created an emotional ride for me as I wondered if this new heart was about to fail to have me go through this physical and emotional pain once again. Ultimately it was determined that I was experiencing rejection, and to address my antibody build-up, the doctors decided I needed a three-part therapy. I found the treatments to be interesting, but I also needed the support of a mental health professional to help me process the multiple levels of grief I was experiencing all at once.

The first treatment is a two-part inpatient process to filter my blood and remove harmful antibodies from my blood plasma, then replace them with antibodies that aren't harmful to my heart. My excitement about the new treatment quickly turned to frustration as I remembered how uncomfortable hospital life could be. I didn't want to spend the weekend in the hospital and was scheduled for another visit after five days. So, against medical advice, I made the knucklehead decision to check out of the hospital. Days after arriving home, some of the side effects of the earlier treatments began to impact me — headache, flushing, chills, wheezing, nausea, and high blood pressure all kicked in.

The morning I was scheduled for "hospital day," my sleep was interrupted by the most painful headache of my life as at 5:00 a.m. In that instant and for the most part of that day, I believed my brain wanted to jump out of my skull. I was readmitted to the hospital. Over the course of the day, this excruciating pain continued with what seemed to be no end in sight. In an instant, I felt relief was coming when I saw the people I affectionately began to call "My Team." My team consisted of the physicians, nurses, and transplant coordinators who took over my transplant care. Every morning I spent in the hospital, they brightened my day when they walked into the room. I found that I depended on them in a way I never expected, as I felt as if these relative strangers actually loved me and would move mountains to care for me. It was after the team showed up the treatments began and the pain began to subside. The level of care I was receiving blew me away; the heart failure team, the infectious disease team, and the neurology team all collaborated to diagnose my new illness. After my first spinal tap, it was determined that I was suffering from non-viral meningitis, a potential result from the earlier treatment. The team treated me for my latest illness, yet I still didn't feel well. What already felt like a never-ending cycle of hospital visits weren't over. Two days after being discharged, I suffered from shortness of breath whenever I was in motion or at rest. My shortness of breath was at such a level that it disturbed the transplant coordinators, and I was asked to return to the hospital for a checkup. We again packed a bag and went back to the hospital. After another heart biopsy, electrocardiogram (EKG), the doctors found that I was now suffering from decreased kidney function and significant dehydration. I spent another few days being treated and was finally at a stable level of health and was able to resume the treatments for rejection.

Throughout the next three days, I received infusions to treat rejection in my tissue. Over the weekend, the transplant clinic was closed, so my Saturday and Sunday treatments were at the cancer center. I was expected to start receiving treatment at the

Winship Cancer Center at Emory on a Sunday morning. it happened to be the fourth day of anti-rejection infusion treatments. This was eye-opening — while my transplant is absolutely a major surgery, seeing all of the people getting chemotherapy and living and fighting various forms of cancer was encouraging.

I don't believe I am exerting myself at a level that should result in fatigue, but all of the procedures were tasking. Once again, I was going to pull back from visitors and increase the amount of rest I was getting. One of the biggest challenges to my healing might have also been one of my biggest blessings. The time between my initial diagnosis to receiving a transplant was only fourteen days. This short timeframe and my health at the time of surgery allowed me to come out of surgery feeling stronger than I assumed to be true for many of those who wait significantly longer. When I was discharged, I felt good. I exceeded all of the goals the medical staff set for me. When they asked me to walk around the floor one time, I walked around twice with strength left over. The doctors would have me do breathing exercises and I would perform at a level beyond expectations. In retrospect, I wished my body was weaker. I wished I wasn't able to leave the hospital and walk a mile and a half. I didn't sufficiently appreciate all that my body and mind had gone through. I wasn't humbled and thought I could walk out of the hospital and return to my normal activity.

The next treatment was really interesting; Belatacept (Bela) that was developed at Emory University Hospital was designed to prevent transplant rejection in adults who have received a kidney transplant. On October 10, 2019, I was the first heart transplant patient in history to receive this treatment at Emory University Hospital. All my life, I never thought I would be the first in relation to anything medically related. The infusion treatment I was taking to combat the rejection I was experiencing left me feeling completely worn out. I entered the room and almost every chair was filled with people who had medicine bags hanging from poles and IV needles in their arms. From my perspective, there appears to be an overwhelming number of young people in the room; however, from Octavia's vantage point, she saw an alarming number of African American males. It is interesting that two people can be in the same space at the same moment and perceive the environment so differently. I analyzed and categorized the room down by age while she did hers by ethnicity, and we both are correct. One thing was certainly true; the patients in this space are there for treatment related to either kidney or heart transplants, and for very few, both organs have been transplanted. The number of African American patients in the hospital at this moment could be attributed to our being in the southeast United States in general or in metropolitan Atlanta in particular. However, the optics underscore African Americans' need for transplants as well as the need for black and brown donors.

13.

"Though one may be overpowered, two can defend themselves. A cord of three strands is not quickly broken."

- Ecclesiastes 4:12 (NIV)

Over time, I have come to agree with my loved ones' opinion that I needed to use the time I have left before I go back to work to rest and rehab. I agreed that I must listen to the doctors and follow their directions. I didn't agree to follow the opinions of my many well-wishers, anyways. I learned that although there are similarities in transplant experiences, which makes support systems so valuable, it is important to have a space to speak your truth without judgment — a space to discuss the changes in you, shared challenges with family, and all that goes on with interpersonal dynamics.

Everyone's experience is different and each has to deal with their own mind in quiet moments. I had hoped to be introduced to a support group that would provide a space to express what was going on with me in a judgment-free zone with others who had similar experiences, not just only to discuss medical issues but to laugh and fellowship. However, my surgeon told me that support groups could be great, but that I should listen only to the medical professionals when it came to health decisions. I was saddened not to have space for support and understanding from individuals with this shared experience, but I hoped to become the thing I longed for through becoming a mentor to future transplant patients through the Georgia Transplant Foundation.

"Cast all your anxiety on him because he cares for you."

- 1 Peter 5:7 (NIV)

There were moments when I told myself that this couldn't possibly be happening to me. It was clear that the transplant was real and I had various scars on my chest as evidence. Yet, with the rejection, the possibility of this new heart failing wasn't possible; it wasn't possible that I would have to relive another heart failing. My denial turned into anger and I began looking for someone or something to blame. My faith in God was in question as to why He let my initial heart failure happen and allowing me to go through this rejection. I was angry with Octavia for not understanding the emotions I was going through; I was blaming her for not being able to make me well with a hug or a word. My anger was irrational but real, and my frustration was directed outward and others undeservingly received my wrath. There were also times when it was focused inward and I did things to physically harm myself. I would either hit myself or not take my medications, knowing that I would be placing myself at risk of relapsing into rejection. As my grief matured, I moved beyond denial to prayer, asking God to turn back the clock and erase my failed heart and the entire experience. I found myself asking Him to make all of this go away so I could return to a better time.

At the time, I had my weekly therapy session with the psychologist. I was proud to have the opportunity to spend time talking about life issues with a qualified professional. Honestly, I was thrilled we found Dr. Parkins and she was so helpful to our family.

Dr. Arthur D. Vaughn

At this time, I longed for some normalcy — something familiar. So, while ill-advised, I went to a meeting for one of the community groups where I was a member. At that point, my home life was tense. Some would say I was contentious, maybe because I was not working and everything was out of balance. My decision irritated Octavia. She was angry and disappointed in me, but I attended the meeting despite her opposition to it. In fact, her behavior often confused me. She made it clear that she intended to dissolve our union, but she continued to care anyway. I would have loved to stay home, but I longed for adult interaction and fellowship. My family had turned into an extension of the nursing staff. When it has something to do with my health, she was an absolute angel; outside of that, she would prefer I stay invisible, so I tried to be just that. Later, I learned that she really wanted me to make my recovery, and by extension, my family, a top priority. From her perspective, my conservatively following the doctor's orders and sitting home in a primarily isolated environment wasn't what she was looking forward for me to do.

Out of these experiences, a couple of realizations became evident. I met with one of the heart failure doctors and she explained the seriousness of my individual situation. While all heart transplant patients are at significant risk for rejection, my risk was higher because my immune system was the initial culprit that infected my heart. I didn't know that my situation created two times as much risk when compared to others, but the risk was higher. The blessing I got was that I was in great hands by getting the best care I could hope for. For my part, I needed to be a great patient, reduce the number of opportunities that will negatively impact my compromised immune system, and rest my body and mind. I was scheduled to return to work and need to do all I can to ensure that when life begins again, I would be ready for it.

While he himself went a day's journey into the wilderness. He came to a broom bush, sat down under it and prayed that he might die. "I have had enough, Lord," he said. "Take my life; I am no better than my ancestors."

- 1 Kings 19:4 (NIV)

Over the course of my recovery, I have had periods of cellular rejection, antibody-mediated rejection, aseptic meningitis, diabetes, acute kidney injury, anxiety, and depression. After my second stint with rejection, the feelings of remorse and anger found their way into the mix of anguish I was already experiencing. I did not understand what was going on and did not know how to manage my feelings. In addition to all I was feeling, I regretted that I had let my marriage fall apart. I was angry that my now estranged wife wouldn't give us another chance. I was frustrated because no one seemed to understand all I was going through.

I was in an agitated state and was looking for relief. One night, I was in the master bathroom engaging in non-suicidal self-injury. I was punching myself in my legs, arms, and chest in an attempt to replace my mental pain with physical pain. My wife walked in and told me to stop. I desperately wanted her to understand what I was going through, but she didn't. She showed no empathy for what I was going through. I would go as far as saying she showed contempt for me at that moment. She was physically present in the household, but I felt abandoned in my mental struggle. I'd been reluctant to say this because of all she has done since my diagnosis, but in reality, she heightened my suffering by announcing her desire for a divorce. I snapped, and the next ten minutes were by far the ugliest moments of our relationship. In every relationship, we have to be careful about what we say and do to our partners.

There are things that can be said and actions you can do that make any hope of reconciliation impossible. I was not certain there was hope for us prior to this night, but after that night, it was clear that our relationship had reached the point of no return.

14.

A lso, there were other nights after this incident where I had given up. I would look at the combination of anti-rejection medications, antidepressants, and sleeping pills in my hand and think I might really be ready to go be with the Lord. There were nights when I did not think I could handle the mental anguish. The mental pain kept me from sleeping at night. I would go up to three days without sleeping, which only made things even worse. During these periods, I would isolate myself from everyone in order to prevent myself from saying or doing things to negatively impact those around me. I would stay in my room with the lights off and under the covers. I found myself eating excessively as a way to find comfort despite my pain.

From time to time, various family members would come and

check in on me and attempt to get me moving, which often didn't come with a good response from me. The help was appreciated, yet I still would not move. Even to this day, I cannot remember the trigger that led to these failures that spiraled into multiple days of depression — and then a new level of depression: Major Depressive Disorder. In truth, I had troubles doing normal day-to-day activities. There were other days when I felt like life wasn't worth living. There were days when I felt as if I was waiting on death to set me free, so two days after my 51st birthday, I wrote a draft of my own obituary and documented my final wishes.

Gracefully Broken

15.

"I have no peace, no quietness; I have no rest, but only turmoil."

- Job 3:26 (NIV)

Mental health is a topic that is attracting more attention but remains a complicated subject. It is my sincere belief that most men internalize what's going on emotionally in an unhealthy way. One in five American adults live with some form of mental illness (National Institute of Mental Health, 2017). The World Health Organization says that one in four people worldwide will experience mental health issues. I believe each of us needs to find a safe space to share our challenges, either with a small group of close friends or through a licensed therapist. I didn't appreciate the emotional toll my heart transplant experience had taken on my psyche, but as the days and months would reveal, the impact was major. Immediately after surgery, I experienced sadness, spontaneous tearfulness, anxiety, self-harm, withdrawal, or irritability. Through therapy, I learned that what I was experiencing is called adjustment disorder. I was responding to the anxiety associated with rapid illness and the associated surgery in ways I did not understand.

During my recovery, I had and continue to experience mood swings, insomnia, and irritability. Through medication, my physicians were working to manage my behavior, so that I don't negatively impact those around me and can get back to a normal life. There were times I would isolate myself when I felt any of the negative feelings coming on, but that is not a long-term solution to my mental illness. I was not always successful and would have to apologize and ask for understanding from those around me. The entire process has been full of ups and downs, and the bad days are really difficult. The surgeries seem to evoke feelings of loss and sorrow, along with opposing feelings of being profoundly moved by feelings of love and gratitude. I believe I see things differently as the old me is dead and gone, but if I am truthful, there are remnants of the ghost of my past that come out, if only for short periods. I have a new perspective on life, and things that were once important to me are now afterthoughts. I still find myself putting up walls and pretending everything is okay in front of family and friends when I am confused or in pain. I know there are people who care about me, but I continue to believe that they simply don't understand what I am going through. I am also still experiencing conflicting feelings that if I share these challenges, I will be perceived as weak. I know I need to move past these old ways of thinking, but breaking these chains is not as easy as others, and I sometimes suggest it is. This is when Man Up needs to mean asking for help!

"If we live, we live for the Lord; and if we die, we die for the Lord. So, whether we live or die, we belong to the Lord.

- Romans 14:8 (NIV)

The twenty-fourth of each month is a day of celebration for me. I celebrate this day as it represents new birth since it is the day my transplant was successfully performed. I've learned that many transplant recipients refer to the day they received their new heart as their second birthday. I wanted to sit outside and see the sunrise without the television or radio on. I could hear the crickets and cicadas. I watched deer move across my neighbor's lawn along with the rare but occasional rabbit. In that moment of peace, I was able to be one with myself and say a prayer of thanksgiving to God. I no longer wanted to be the man that holds in all of his emotions. I've learned that when I hold in my emotions, they eventually come out in a non-constructive manner. I felt the pain in my chest and have to remember that what I am feeling isn't my old heart, but my sternum healing after it was cracked open during surgery. I often forgot I have a new heart and wasn't anticipating the feeling that came before my old heart needed to be shocked into a normal rhythm.

At night, when it is quiet and I am alone, I experienced and continue to experience nightmares that wake me up calling for help. I used to experience angry outbursts, but those happen infrequently now, nonetheless I am also aware that they can happen. The time alone — when I have nothing but my thoughts to comfort me — is when I feel the most vulnerable. It is at night that I usually feel as if the chemical balance in my mind is off-balance and my brain is floating inside my head. I've been given a drug that seems to balance out those feelings, but

I'm yet to understand why this is happening. I fear that I may be overmedicated with one drug that is intended to manage my emotions by day, and others that help me sleep at night. I feel increasingly distant from people who I would have once considered closest to me.

A rush of regret and emotion flowed over me like a tidal wave because I lived at the expense of another, and I began to cry uncontrollably. I went through the physical pain, but the emotional pain seems to be endless. I can't help but wonder if the plan is to torment my soul or make me pay for misdeeds. The anxiety, depression, sadness, and crying I routinely experienced are all traits and behaviors I believed were associated with weak people. I believed that those around me did not understand what I was going through and would see me differently. My sense was that my family would see me as a weak person and no longer as the protector and provider I once was. Interestingly, I don't believe I am the only one who views the display of these emotions as a sign of weakness. I knew I was different, the pain in my chest was no longer there, but I remember the sense of frailty and vulnerability were at the top of my mind.

It's been said that the short time from my diagnosis to

transplant is an evidence that God has a plan for my life. There is not a day that goes by when I don't ask myself, *what is God's grand plan for my life?* I question why He didn't just let me die when I initially became ill, or while in the theatre. Now I have this second chance, and the question of what I am supposed to do with it continues to dominate my thoughts. Clearly, not doing something significant with the new opportunity at life would dishonor the gift. But the pressing question that has yet to be answered is: "Why me?"

Since the transplant, I have melted down a number of times. Initially, the breakdown centered on "Why me?" I couldn't and haven't processed why I am still alive after my heart failed. Out of everyone on earth, why was I granted unmerited favor and why did someone else have to pass away so I could live? Another family, and community, was grieving while we were celebrating life. Then I have this second chance, and what am I supposed to do with it? These breakdowns come with strong emotional responses; I break down in fits of shaking, crying, and dysfunction. There are times when I have felt that my wife should have just let me die instead of working on getting me the transplant. I've been having issues ever since the surgery, and it's been suggested that I was suffering from depression prior to becoming ill, and afterward, it only worsened. I resumed seeing a therapist that I had worked with previously, and the transplant team prescribed antidepressants to help with the issues I was experiencing. I was spiraling downward and was engaging in non-suicidal self-injury, finding myself remaining in bed in a dark room and engaging in emotional eating that led to dramatic fluctuations in my weight.

As a result of my disturbing statements and erratic behavior, I found myself back at Emory, this time for a twenty-four-hour psychiatric admission. Upon my arrival, I was given a room in the cardiac care unit. I saw many familiar faces, which put me at ease. After the check-in process, a psychiatrist joined me, and we talked about what I was feeling and thinking. I was struggling with the trauma of the transplant, the dissolution of my marriage, and the effects of all the medicine I was taking. I was sleep-deprived and felt a sense of isolation within me. There would be periods when I would not sleep for up to three days and then crash. We agreed that I would stay the night for observation. The nursing staff went into stealth mode and was able to remove all the cords and sharp objects from my room without my notice. They also made sure anything in the bag I brought with me couldn't be used to harm others or myself.

Prior to being checked in, I locked my handgun in its safe and gave the safe to my attorney for safekeeping. I never considered shooting myself or anyone else, but I never thought I would get so depressed that I needed to be admitted to the hospital for a psychiatric stay either. I am a firm believer in responsible gun ownership, but the last thing I would ever want to do is hurt someone when I was in an altered mental state.

During my stay, there was a nurse assigned to me who literally watched me for the twenty-four hours duration — she would sit there while I was asleep, watching television, or doing a crossword puzzle. Occasionally, we would chat about what was on television and other random thoughts. She helped when I needed my blood pressure checked, when I needed blood drawn for labs, and when I needed other assorted things taken care of. It was a very interesting night, and I enjoyed being back in the hospital during this time. Being in the hospital had become a familiar space, and there was always someone there willing to talk to me, which was in direct contrast to the isolation I felt when I was at home. After the twenty-four hours stay, it was determined that I was not a threat to others or myself, and I was discharged. An outcome of my stay was a diagnosis that my adjustment disorder had transitioned to

Major Depressive Disorder (MDD).

MDD disorder does not discriminate — impacting roughly twelve-and-a-half percent of all races, ages, and socio-economic backgrounds. (Trivedi Madhukar, H., 2008). Working with a psychiatrist based at the hospital and an independent therapist, I was able to receive treatment in the form of depression-focused psychotherapy along with drug therapy. As I began to gradually improve, I worked with both doctors to develop strategies to maintain emotional stability, which included self-care activities, such as playing golf, bike riding, and walking. Each one of these activities was a physical struggle, but focused my mind and helped my body to regain strength.

As I moved through the healing process, I learned why my loved ones were trying to get me to slow down, rest, and allow myself to heal. I now understand that I still hadn't allowed myself to mentally process the trauma of becoming so ill so fast, believing I had died, and working through the concept of favor and why I am here. I learned that being home was emotionally unhealthy for me. While I am fortunate that Octavia was caring for me, the atmosphere associated with our relationship created a fractured mental state in me. I don't blame her for anything because my actions or inaction created the situation in which I found myself in. I have noticed that the emotional outbursts and insomnia I experienced at home are non-existent when I am in the hospital. Being home is impeding my progress.

I never imagined that the person who has been the rudder in my life and best friend for over two decades would be a deterrent to my mental and physical well-being. I believe this sudden realization may become helpful in my recovery process and a point of discussion when I see my therapist. There continued to be strings of days when I didn't sleep for forty-eight to seventy-two hours at a time. There are other days when I am unable to get out of bed, and I would sit in a dark room by myself lost in depression. When I do sleep, I usually struggle to sleep through the night, and I find myself experiencing persistent fear, and when I wake up I'd feel like I am suffocating. There are other times when I appear to wake up, but am not fully conscious and I'd see myself throwing punches that would make Mike Tyson proud. I am not sure if I am fighting an invisible enemy or fighting my own gremlins. After a few minutes, I would climb back into bed and fall asleep.

My therapist, Dr. Parkins, said that I couldn't run from my gremlins. I have to face them head-on. For me, a highly functioning person suffering from depression can be compared to a highly functioning alcoholic. The depressed person and the alcoholic are similar in that they are both able to perform daily activities, attend work, or participate in children's activities and other engagements, all while masking the anxiety, self-doubt, and feeling of not being enough. This is why having a small group of champions I can call when experiencing this would be helpful, and it's been suggested that using breathing exercises, writing, and prayer can be beneficial when anxious moments begin to take over me. I have to embrace this life change and really begin changing my lifestyle. These last twenty-four hours has to be something I should take to heart. I have to change. I have to rest! I have to create a new reality for myself.

I didn't know how to deal with the mountain of emotions that I was feeling, and this resulted in harming myself. As mentioned earlier, I would literally beat myself — punching myself so hard that I would bruise my body, and at times, even break the skin and cause bleeding. The physical pain I would cause myself was extreme, but a fitting substitute for the mental pain. Most often, people associate this behavior with teenagers cutting themselves, scratching, banging, hitting, or biting themselves. I didn't know that what I was doing had a name, but I was doing it just the same. I was prescribed drugs to help regulate my mood, but they often don't work. When I am driving, I often find myself pulling the car over to cry and feel like I am on an emotional rollercoaster. Through the course of treatment, the therapist concluded that I am suffering from a high functioning depression and was struggling with non-suicidal self-injury. It has become very apparent that the doctors were able to repair my body, but this experience also shattered my mind.

"Scorn has broken my heart and has left me helpless; I looked for sympathy, but there was none, for comforters, but I found none."

- Psalm 69:20 (NIV)

There were nights when I would cry myself to sleep. There were days during my various periods of hopelessness when I would reach out to close friends seeking support. I don't have a sense that they knew or shared the depths of what I was feeling. There were times when I attempted to share what I was feeling with my now estranged wife. While she witnessed everything that occurred during my illness, she didn't appear to understand the toll my illness, my recovery, and our home life was having on me, and it became a burden too heavy to bear alone. There was an instance when she and I were in the car running errands, and one of our many conflicts reared its ugly head. I don't remember what we were arguing about, and it clearly wasn't important, but instead of having that shouting match, I jumped out of the moving car and walked two miles back to the house. My actions infuriated her because from her point of view, I was constantly fighting against her when she was trying to ensure I did and ate the right things.

After being out one evening, something snapped in my mind, and I became unhinged. I left the house at 2:30 a.m. with no destination in mind. I just knew that I wanted to be somewhere else. I drove around for hours going nowhere and ended up parking in a Waffle House parking lot. I cried for a while, questioned my sanity, grabbed a blanket that I brought with me, and went to sleep. I wasn't sure what was going on, but I decided that I needed to get away. At that moment, living or dying didn't matter; I just wanted my gremlins to go away. I wanted what I was feeling to end and didn't care how. This was a dangerous time for me. I pray that others understand there are options that I didn't realize were available to me at that time. I came to my senses enough to call a friend of thirty years. After my fifth call, following spending the night in my truck, he answered. He was out of town, but I always have had access to his home. He was worried about me and told me to go over to his home and not to sleep in the street. I realized that I didn't have my wallet or any cash, so not only was I driving without a license, I didn't have the means to get anything to eat, and my medications were at home. Thank God for rideshare food services. . . I was able to utilize the app on my phone to get some food that afternoon. I reached out to another friend, and she talked me off the ledge. However, without my medicine, I was becoming increasingly ill. Yet, for the moment, I did not care.

I still don't know how, but I arrived back home the next evening very weak, bewildered, and with a temperature over one hundred degrees. I walked into an empty home, drained, and in need of a shower. I cleaned myself up and climbed in the bed vulnerable, still confused, and clearly not concerned about my health. After speaking with the transplant coordinators, I got back on my medications, rested and physically returned to the healing process. My next move was to begin to work on healing my mind. I reached out to the therapist that I had seen bi-weekly since being initially discharged from the hospital. Dr. Parkins and I doubled the frequency in which we were meeting.

Later, my psychiatrist adjusted the dosage of the medication that was intended to restore the chemical balance in the brain.

Life will be brighter than noonday, and darkness will become like morning. You will be secure, because there is hope; you will look about you and take your rest in safety.

- Job 11:17-19 (NIV)

Everyone who reads this should be assured that there is hope. Mental health challenges are not limited to a single race, color, gender, or identity. Women are twice as likely to be diagnosed with depression compared with men (Hasin, Goodwin, Stinson, et al., 2005). However, women are four times less likely to commit suicide than men (Oquendo, Ellis, Greenwald, et al., 2001). Caucasian Americans are diagnosed with Major Depressive Disorder at a higher rate than African Americans. Regrettably, African Americans resist treatment and suffer longer and struggle longer than our White peers (Williams, Gonzalez Neighbors, Nesse, Abelson, Sweetman, & Jackson 2007).

From speaking with my male peers, I understood that many believe that acknowledging a mental health condition is a sign of weakness or some sort of punishment from God. In fact, depressed men of color underutilize mental health professionals, which is a contributing factor to our having the highest mortality rate of any ethnic/racial group in the United States (Hankerson, Suite & Bailey, 2015). Similar to how some address physical health, masculine norms, and the overall underutilization of health services led men to not taking advantage of healthcare services. Research suggests that there are socio-cultural factors such as racism and discrimination, mistrust of health care providers, misdiagnosis, and clinician bias that contribute to African American men's resistance to seeking assistance with depression disorder (Hankerson, Suite & Bailey, 2015).

Despite efforts like those of nonprofit groups like 'Silence the Shame' to normalize the conversation around mental health, men are significantly less likely to seek help compared with depressed women (Hammond, 2012). I am clearly not a therapist or here to give advice, but I will share how I recovered.

I experienced a revolving door of therapists. I could not open up and did not trust any of them. I was unwilling to share deep secrets with them for fear of being vulnerable. I've met with a number of people over the years, and it can be challenging to find one you bond with. This experience is a bond like Adam and Eve in Genesis 2:25; you have to be emotionally naked and not ashamed. If we are willing to seek help, each of us can recover from anxiety and depression.

I sought out someone who was culturally competent. Cultural competence is used to describe the therapist's ability to understand how your philosophies, principles, values, and beliefs are aligned with theirs. This is not to suggest that one has to find a mental health professional of their own race, gender, or similar socio-economic level. I am suggesting it's about someone who appreciates these things and can empathize when treating you as their patient. I believe you have to find someone who can acknowledge their own biases and see past them. I once met with a therapist who coincidently was a woman. Through the first three sessions, it became evident to me that she had a level of fear that prevented us from connecting. Whether this fear was racial bias or not, I do not know, but that fear prevented me from developing a level of trust with her, and our sessions ended. This is not to say men can't work with female therapists; in fact, I love my therapist, who happens to be a woman. It seems to me that several therapists I met with did not understand how men express depression. My experience suggests that when a therapist isn't sensitive to the patient's accumulated life experiences and their impact, it can lead to misdiagnoses or the wrong treatment plan. My therapist was critical to my recovery, which only came after she was able to break through the walls I created. I was able to receive comments that I sometimes didn't want to hear about myself after we developed a trusting relationship. We met weekly, and it took months before I opened up and became transparent with her.

Another challenge I faced was trying to reach out to my friends and family. Your social circle can be a help or hindrance to your recovery (Galdas, Cheater, Marshall, 2005). I do believe that they care for me as I do for them. However, they have no training, and if they haven't gone through a depressive episode, their well-intended psychoanalysis is often off base and can be more harmful than helpful. I've tried to get a sense of how others in my social circle perceive depression. There are periods when I wanted to reach out to someone between sessions with my physiatrist or therapist, but refrained because I simply didn't think anyone would understand. In these moments, I found myself suffering alone. Through therapy, I found that I became more in touch with my feelings in a permanent way.

Depression, like cardiovascular disease and hypertension, can be a silent killer if gone undiagnosed and untreated.

"But the Advocate, the Holy Spirit, whom the Father will send in my name, will teach you all things and will remind you of everything I have said to you."

- John 14:26 (NIV)

After meeting with various therapists from a variety of races, both male and female, I found a person who has been able to break the chains that Job describes in chapter 36:8 — that bound people through affliction. I have learned a great deal about myself through therapy, but it took some time for me to become open to the process. The process offers a supportive environment and allows you to be more honest with yourself than you may have ever been. Most people who know me would be surprised to learn that I had self-esteem issues. My self-doubt is a double-edged sword that fueled my success, but it was also a destructive force. Through this process, I began to explore how my upbringing partly shaped how I viewed friendships and familiar relationships. As we explored who I was at the core, long-buried post-traumatic stress was kicked loose.

In addition to anxiety and depression coming to the forefront of post-surgery, I have long dealt with defeating self-doubt where I doubt myself and all that I've accomplished. My therapist has suggested that I suffer from having a low level of self-esteem that I mask through arrogance. My outward-facing life would suggest that I have it together—the wall of awards, proclamations, photos with celebrities, and dignitaries. In reality, this "Imposter Syndrome" contributes too much of the anxiety that keeps me up at night. However, this same fear of failure creates a duality that also drives me to achieve professional and academic success.

Over the days and months to follow, I had to continue to work toward returning to myself. My measuring stick remained what I thought I was prior to the illness. The norm during my childhood was to have both parents in the household, and my image of a man was instilled in me by my father. I perceived myself as this superhero. I was a strong man that financially provided and physically protected my family. My weapon was my mind, and if needed physically, my size and demeanor could at least make someone think twice before threatening my family or me. Growing up in New York, there were times when physical prowess was a desirable trait. I am not sure that I was everything I thought I was prior to my falling ill. Nor had I accepted the realization that each of us who go through a traumatic process will have to travel part of this course alone. After surgery, I felt emotionally and physically weak. My body failed me for the first time, and I questioned if I would ever recover.

Just as we need to deal with our physical health, we must also take proper care of our emotional and mental health. After exploring who and why I am, we were able to address how I was handling the anxiety and depression that I was experiencing. In therapy, I also gained a greater understanding of those things that trigger certain behaviors when I experienced extreme instances of stress and uncomfortable emotions. I also acquired a profound appreciation for the role that caregivers and medical professionals play in the healing process. I also learned that there are quiet moments when each of us will deal with the despair that comes with remorse.

"You must act according to the decisions they give you at the place the Lord will choose. Be careful to do everything they instruct you to do."

- Deuteronomy 17:10 (NIV)

We are taught that God's light is either enlarged or diminished by the decisions we make. In hindsight, I believe that I was living a life that would be considered unacceptable in God's sight. I wasn't all bad, and I did many good things in service to others, but in a final evaluation, I was not living a life that would be pleasing in His sight. I grew up in the church, being active at varying levels over the years. But through my period of healing, my relationship with my Lord and Savior became stronger.

I remember some years back when a friend reportedly died from a self-inflicted gunshot wound. The memory of the death of my friend has stayed with me ever since then, and in part, kept me from causing harm to myself. I spoke to family members who encouraged me to continue to work with my therapist. I was reminded that death is final, and while my marriage had fallen apart, I still have daughters who need their father. I was reminded that God's hands were in play for my life to be saved, and that He is not done with me yet. I was reminded that He has a plan for me. Now, I wouldn't want to mislead anyone to believing that prayer and gospel music were the tools that got me back to my right mind, nor would I want to suggest that they were not a significant part of my recovery

— the messages in the music and the laying of my issues on the altar of prayer lifted burdens from my mind and gave me some measure of tranquility. However, in addition to my renewed walk with God, we also added a psychiatrist to augment my mental health team that already included a licensed professional counselor.

Over the months, my mental disposition had improved through a combination of prayer, therapy, and medication. There had been no end to my journey towards mental health. Every day I wake up praying that it's going to be a good day. Every day I wake up hoping to be fully functional. There are days when I feel like my old self, but that rarely lasts for a full day. Make no mistake, there are days when I fight with myself to get out of the bed, there are days when I fight with myself to have a productive day, and there are others when I don't get out of bed at all. There is no magic wand to feeling better. I feel as if the best thing I can do is work with the mental health providers in order to find the tools to manage my various mental health crises allowing me to be self-sufficient.

After working through some of my emotional issues, I attempted to test my physical condition by playing golf. Golf is a game that requires a lot of focus and technique in order to be successful. My game could not have been much worse. I attempted fifteen of the eighteen holes for the round. I found my body failing and experienced dizziness and weakness in my extremities. I found that I could not focus on the game, and it showed in my play. I don't think the experience could have been any less enjoyable. Thankfully, I was playing with friends who never get frustrated when one of the group plays poorly. I think we were harder on ourselves than our friends were on us. After playing golf, I was exhausted and slept in the passenger seat for pretty much the entire hour ride home. For the balance of the day, the effects of this were evident. I believe learning my limits was an important part of my healing process.

After six months of worrying that my body was not accepting my new heart, I was now experiencing no rejection. My new heart was functioning well for the moment. I could resume working toward healing and focus on being stable. Until I began to recover mentally, the physical healing could not begin. There are times when I feel that the high number of medications had more control of this body than I did. I had to recognize that the healing doesn't have a defined end date, and I need to be patient and let it happen in its own time. It is my hope that my journey can be a source of hope and inspiration for others. I am patiently waiting to see what His plans are for me.

My Testimony

16.

Do not be anxious about anything, but in every situation, by prayer and petition, with thanksgiving, present your requests to God. And the peace of God, which transcends all understanding, will guard your hearts and your minds in Christ Jesus.

- Philippians 4:6-7 (NIV)

Yesterday, I sat on a stage with cardiovascular medical and research experts in front of several hundred people discussing about heart health. The people who attended were successful in their own transplant surgeries and likely looked at me as same. Little did they know that while on stage, I was experiencing impostor syndrome. For those who don't know what impostor syndrome is, it's a pattern in which someone doubts their accomplishments and has a persistent internalized fear of being exposed as a "fraud." When we were done many of those in attendance visited with me expressing their gratitude for my willingness to share such a person story. Later we received amazing feedback saying it was one of the best Men's Healthy Heart Breakfasts to date.

Over the course of treatment, I learned that this self-doubt is not uncommon with people in general, and as a result of life experience, various microaggressions can impact how we perceive ourselves. These intentional or unintentional verbal, behavioral, and environmental indignities communicate hostile, derogatory, or negative racial slights and insults to a member of a differing racial group (Sue, Nadal, Capodilupo, Lin, Torino, & Rivera, 2008). During our weekly meetings, we explored my feelings of anxiety, depression, sleep difficulties, and an overall lack of confidence.

While it takes time to unpack root causes of these feelings, being open to acknowledging that these things exist and being willing to talk about them is critical to the recovery process. It wasn't until after my transplant surgery and the devastating post-surgery emotional trauma that I began to acknowledge that these issues were far-reaching in my life. Others have found that having a sense of internal excellence and validation serve as successful protective mechanisms. I have, as well as others, used shifting as a coping mechanism when dealing with racial microaggressions. Simply put, shifting is strategically emphasizing common experiences and interests shared with our White colleagues, and de-emphasizing racial and ethnic differences as a way to avoid being viewed as the spokesperson for all African Americans (Franklin, 1999).

17.

"He who finds a wife finds what is good and receives favor from the Lord."

- Proverbs 18:22 (NIV)

Family is tough, and mine was no different. June 19, 2019, marked twenty years of marriage for us. From the outside looking in, we had a great marriage. We met thirty years ago while we were students at Syracuse University. We literally had the white house in the suburbs — no picket fence, but we did have two kids and a dog. We had it all! She was heavily involved in the church, and I was in leadership positions in a variety of community organizations. Like many of us, we see people through the lens of social media where we usually see a snapshot of a person's life versus the collage of experiences that comprise the totality of a person's experiences.

Our kids are relatively well behaved, academically successfully, and attend church regularly. We both have solid careers, take wonderful vacations, and rub elbows with Atlanta's elite at various galas and social functions. Like any relationship, we have had our shares of ups and downs. I will admit that I am where I am today because of my wife's support and sacrifice.

He went on: "What comes out of a person is what defiles them. For it is from within, out of a person's heart, that evil thoughts come—sexual immorality, theft, murder, adultery, greed, malice, deceit, lewdness, envy, slander, arrogance and folly. All these evils come from inside and defile a person."

- Mark 7:20-23 (NIV)

Through the ups and downs of the last two decades, my estranged wife had been the compass that kept #TeamVaughn moving in the right direction. She was the primary parent in the raising of our two wonderful girls, and allowed me to pursue my dreams while loving me during my many mistakes. As I mentioned earlier, she rarely left my side from diagnoses, through my stay in the hospital, and during the early part of my recovery at home. I will also value her for carrying the entire load during my illness. As I will discuss later, the responsibilities of the caregiver weigh heavily on them and are often overlooked.

On August 29, 2019, it all came crumbling down when my wife made it abundantly clear that our marriage was officially over. I had not done all of the things described in Mark 7:20-23, but my life and attitude certainly reflected a number of them. I had become prideful and arrogant and stopped going to church; I behaved as if the various titles I held put me above others. I treated the woman I had pursued in college and asked to marry me over two decades ago with disdain for no reason. I stayed out late regularly, neglecting my kids, and my responsibilities. The medical diagnosis may have been acute heart failure, but I believe my heart had become hard over the years, and it began to die because I dishonored all that I should have treasured.

I would engage in various forms of self-medication that, at times, included smoking cigars to soothe my mind and drinking excessively, which was an abnormal behavior for me. I would also avoid my situation at home by not coming home until very late, and then getting up in the morning and going to activities. I learned that this behavior started a downward cycle that led to my wife and kids feeling abandoned, and they withdrew from me. In turn, I began feeling a heightened sense of loneliness. Our relationship splintered to the point where our marriage counselor told us that we both had been behaving more like roommates than a married couple. The counselor went as far as to say that we were living separate lives under the same roof. I am hoping to be a cautionary tale for other couples. Go to your spouse, who I pray is your best friend, and share your gremlins with them and attempt to work through them together. When you are have having issues — spiritual, emotional, financial, or other — lay them on the altar and seek God's help.

She was the rock I leaned on and the stable person in my life. While we were having issues prior to my falling ill, many of which I was the source or a contributing factor to, the timing of her announcement and the harsh behavior she had privately displayed was wrecking my emotions. Publicly, she was displaying a model of care and love for her husband, who has fallen ill. She doesn't want people to know our situation because she doesn't want anyone to think she left me during my time of need. Privately, she showed great disdain for me, having few words other than contempt, and her bitterness was like I've never seen. She has become increasingly hardened yet is still very caring. Her behavior adds to my confusion and emotional instability.

Despite our relationship status, we remained cordial and made sure the other was well. One night while out to get some food, she shared a song with me, "My Testimony" by Marvin Sapp. I am and have been a believer in the Holy Trinity all of my life. This song moved me, brought emotions out of me that I never knew were in me, from the Holy Spirit. Tears flowed from my eyes, my body shook, and my hands were raised to the sky. I danced in a way I've only seen others do when they are in God's presence. I've not understood and dare say I was skeptical when seeing someone "catch the Holy Spirit." I've questioned if it was for show or attention, but today what I experienced confirmed that it's not. I felt like I had a spiritual breakthrough. This was the exact opposite of the mental breakdowns I've been experiencing. Instead of tearing me down mentally, the song uplifted my spirit, thereby bringing a smile and positive energy to my soul. The spirit of God was here tonight. Following the first song, we listened to "More Than I Can Bear" by God's

Property. Writing this down doesn't fully translate, and doesn't do justice to what happened to me. The Spirit of God was there that night. It was a moment of pure praise — when you go to God asking Him for nothing, but giving Him praise and thanks. A sense of comfort flowed over me during this period that I could only attribute to the Holy Spirit.

As I continue to think of the separation and eventual divorce between my wife and me, I can't paint this season as all good or all bad. If anything, I would describe this time as contradictory. Right now, I need to focus on how to manage my emotions. When the stress from my health issues or the underlying stress of our marriage comes to the forefront, I need non-medicated tools to help manage the feelings. It's been suggested using breathing exercises, writing, prayer, and gym time as the regimen. I have to embrace this life change and really begin changing my lifestyle. I have to change. I had to rest! I had to create a new reality for myself. I experienced something like I never experienced before. This could only be God's hand on my life. Man Up has to mean loving your wife as Christ loves His church.

18.

"Therefore what God has joined together, let no one separate."

- Mark 10:9 (NIV)

The month after surgery, I began to feel what I termed survivors remorse. Over the months that followed, there were many sleepless nights with multiple occasions going as long as thirty-six hours without sleep. I often felt irritated or vulnerable, which caused my mind to work overtime. These breaks came with strong emotional responses; I broke down in fits of shaking, crying, and become dysfunctional. I think these feelings became enhanced since my wife notified me that she wanted a divorce. We were having issues prior to my falling ill, but a combination of the trauma I experienced and the medications I was taking animated all of my responses. There were times over the course of my healing when I felt like my estranged wife hated me or took pleasure in my pain. Later, I learned that she did not draw pleasure from my pain. In fact, she hadn't figured out how to process her own pain while caring for me at the same time.

There are a couple of things I needed to remember when feeling that way, the first being that we are estranged for a reason. While everyone has some fault in a failed relationship, I have to take more than fifty percent of the fault in this one. I am sure her feelings of alienation came with the belief that I am ninety percent or more at fault. So, when I feel she enjoys my suffering, it is partially self-pity and partially my failure to recognize her pain, her feeling of betrayal, and her unwillingness to be vulnerable and risk being hurt by me again.

There were days when I felt run down, but I managed. I did find myself becoming emotional from time to time. I can't help but think that many feelings may have been a result of my meeting with my attorney today. We spent time this afternoon discussing and drafting a large part of the proposed divorce agreement. We've talked about it before, but now it was more than just talk. The payment of the retainer and drafting of the proposal makes it all real. Someone once said, "It's one thing to ask for a divorce. It's another thing to file for one."

If I am honest, I feel my pending divorce is more of a driving force in my downward spin. The various medical professionals I met with agreed — the trauma of the illness, surgery, the dissolution of our relationship along with multiple rejections, were creating mental stress that would negatively impact the strongest of minds. The post-surgery feelings would be there, but everything is heightened by having to go through this alone. I wish we could get this divorce settled, and I would then get my own place and move forward. The cohabitating is mentally straining. I think one way or the other, I needed to move out. The breakup itself is off-putting, but then I never know which wife I am going to get, the one who can't stand to look at me or the one who is going to show compassion and caring. It's taken a moment, but beyond my denial that there is hope for us, I see how she truly wants no interaction with me. She will say things with venom, like: "You need to learn to care for yourself." She will do things to ensure that she and our minor daughter are taken care of and leave me to fend for myself, which is historically an uncommon act. The harshness in her tone and general unwillingness to engage with me often triggered mental episodes. In the past, I dealt with issues like this by putting up a wall. I would become distant, show anger, and respond with my own meanness. I am not that person anymore. I am unable to function in that manner; I don't want to be that person.

Good or bad, it's been the longest relationship I've had. Despite all of our challenges, we would always come back to one another, and when the push came to shove, we were going to have each other's back. As much as I loved her, I continued to mourn the death of our relationship. I need to get the paperwork completed and treat this separation like a business transaction and prepare to move on. I have to accept the reality that any love she once had for me is either gone or buried under miles of bitterness. We need to move on and figure out how to live and love ourselves again, and forgive ourselves. This process has taken longer than I ever thought it would, and I am uncertain why. Some have suggested that she may be having second thoughts. While that may be true, I believe that we both have said and done things that would make reconciliation an impossible mission. As time passed, I became more at peace with the decision for us to break up. A friend shared this pearl of wisdom with me: "She is a good person but may no longer be the right person for you." I believe it is time for us to move on without each other as this relationship has taken its course.

"I cannot carry all these people by myself; the burden is too heavy for me."

- Numbers 11:14 (NIV)

The weight on the caregivers of chronically ill patients is often overlooked. Through this process, I have learned that long-term caregivers are at higher risk for cardiovascular disease, substantially due to increased physical, emotional, or financial burdens resulting from their increased need to provide support to a family member. According to the National Alliance for Caregiving (2005), caregivers share the pains of patients, often requiring additional attention and support due to the demands and pressure. During my experience with serious illness, I witnessed that caregiving was not limited to a specific generation, income or educational level, or racial group. As I sat in the hospital, I watched families walk by the door, experiencing the stress of caring for a loved one, while often disregarding their own needs. I also learned about the physical, emotional, and financial strain that a major unexpected illness could cause for both the patient and caregiver. According to the

Capistrant, B. D., Moon, J. R., Berkman, L. F., & Glymour, M. M. (2012), long-term caregivers often have more health issues than people who haven't had similar experiences.

Due to the attention I required, my primary caregiver's longstanding exercise routine diminished. We watched her level of fatigue increase along with the return of significant concerns with hypertension. This is particularly concerning as Barnes, Schneider, Alexander, & Staggers (1997) noted that cardiovascular disease resulting from untreated or poorly managed hypertension is the leading cause of death for African Americans. Forty-five percent of African American women die from cardiovascular-related illnesses. This exceeds the percentage of deaths from all other causes, including cancer, stroke, and diabetes. According to a report released by caregiving.org, six of ten caregivers are women with many finding purpose and meaning in their roles as caregivers. I don't know that my primary caregiver found purpose or meaning in this role, but she took the role seriously and ensured that the coordination with the medical team pre- and post-transplant was taken care of in a loving and professional manner.

There is another group of caregivers that we don't discuss enough, known as the "Sandwich Generation." Unlike baby boomers, Generation X, Millennial or Generation Z, the Sandwich Generation isn't defined by the year you were born. The Sandwich Generation includes those who are caring for both children and ailing parents. A 2020 article by The Pew Research Center states that roughly twelve-and-a-half percent of Americans between the ages of forty and sixty are members of this so-called Sandwich generation. As more and more people of my generation became members of the Sandwich Generation, I've learned that we are being expected to perform tasks that I expected my skilled nurses to carry out like injections, feedings, catheter, colostomy care, and other difficult procedures.

19.

Honor your father and your mother, as the Lord your God has commanded you, so that you may live long and that it may go well with you in the land the Lord your God is giving you.

- Deuteronomy 5:16 (NIV)

I never had the blessing of experiencing caring for my parents and children at the same time. My mother passed away two months before my 27th birthday. My dad passed away a few years later in 2000 when I was thirty-one. My daughters were never able to meet and get to know their paternal grandparents. This is something that was clearly outside of my control, but it is an experience I wish they had. I learned so much from my maternal grandparents that I wished they had that opportunity. Fortunately, they are able to regularly spend time with their maternal grandmother.

During my illness, I realized how unprepared we were regarding plans for any long-term care I potentially would require. We didn't have a plan on how we would meet our normal and any long-term financial responsibilities. I hadn't communicated my desires related to health care decisions. I also learned that the position we were in was more common than I knew. As a result, I've made sure to document my wishes regarding health decisions in case I can't make them myself, and who should make them on my behalf. I reviewed my life insurance policies to confirm the amount I had, and who the beneficiaries are. As I write this, I am working with an attorney to draft a will to make sure everything is handled in case of my untimely demise. We never know the day and time when we will leave this planet, but one thing is sure — it will happen to each of us. I learned that securing life insurance is considerably more difficult after a major illness; I was fortunate that I already had that in place. However, far too many of us don't plan for that day when we will pass away, and we then rely on crowd-funding to pay our burial expenses. Far too many of us haven't planned for our loved ones to be provided for when our life comes to an end.

As you read this, I encourage you to secure a life insurance policy in addition to the one you may have with your employer. I ask that you meet with an attorney and draft a will. Wills are not only for the wealthy, but they allow you to decide the disposition of your possessions on your own terms.

My family dynamics is difficult and really is an outgrowth of my upbringing. My late father was a complicated man of his time and circumstance, which taught me some of the concepts of manhood I still hold dearly to this day. He also provided examples of what I should not be as a man. My father grew up in Murfreesboro, Tennessee, in a circumstance where neither of his parents wanted him. My paternal grandfather, Clarence, was born on April 19, 1905, in Rockvale, Tennessee — a rural section of the state just eleven miles from Murfreesboro. Granddad Clarence provided a weak example of family and manhood, and in my estimation, this example, in part, shaped my father's thinking as he grew into adulthood. My paternal grandmother, Sally Mae Blackmon, left the family early in my father's life, and he had inconsistent contact with her until he was eighteen. After completing the ninth grade, my father left school and opted for work until he was old enough to enlist in the United States Army.

Dr. Arthur D. Vaughn

My father, Sergeant Alfred McKinley Vaughn, Sr., was one of the men who helped change the role African Americans played in the military. Men like my father ended up in the northern states as a part of the great migration where African Americans fled the oppression and racism of the southern states seeking a better life in the northern urban areas between 1916 and 1970. Many of these men ended up in civil service or blue-collar jobs after serving in the military during the Korean or Vietnam wars. Prior to the Korean War, less than eight percent of the approximately 1,250,000 members of the United States Armed Forces were African American. My father served with distinction during the Korean War (1950 – 1953). He was awarded four Bronze Stars for combat heroism and meritorious service. Moreover, he was awarded the Korean Service Medal for participation in the Korean War, the Army of Occupation Medal for service while assigned to Germany, and the United Nations Service Medal; the first international award ever created by the United Nations which recognized those who participated in the Korean War to ensure the protection of South Korea. Based on his separation papers (DD-214), my father was honorably discharged from the United States Army in August of 1953. The Korean War changed the face of the American military. According to the Veterans Administration, this was the first time African Americans served side by side in the same units with service members of all races, and were afforded the opportunity to lead in combat.

Despite my father's complex background, he always provided for his family. One thing our father taught us was to look out for each other. I remember after being taught that public assistance is a bridge for those who have fallen on hard times, my dad further taught me that when you have seven siblings, you are each other's public assistance. My father and the men in the community I grew up in were providers! After my dad's military service ended, he elected to move to New York City with his mother instead of returning to rural Murfreesboro, Tennessee. Over the next nineteen years, my father had eight children from three women — he had two sons prior to meeting and marrying my mother, Gregory and Mark; and then after he married my mother Delores, there were five kids: Adrienne, Alfred, Andrew, Aretha, and me; Arthur. My father also had a child during a period while my parents were separated, Kenneth.

My father spent the majority of his work life serving as a sanitation employee for the City of New York. He coached the youth football and served as a little league baseball coach and umpire. He instilled a work ethic and strength of character in me. My dad could not provide everything for us that we desired, but we had everything we needed. He worked one and sometimes three jobs to ensure we had a roof over our heads and food on our table. As long as the work was legal, he didn't mind doing it . . . no matter how difficult. He and the other men in the community served as mentors and role models for the boys in the neighborhood, and to this day, it brings a smile to my face when my peers from home tell stories about what my father meant to them. When I see the kids I grew up with now serving as the coaches in my hometown, I can't help but think that the men we grew up with, including my father, are still present in the community.

I believe my father instilled a sense of community in me, teaching me to serve the community and mentor young men who weren't fortunate enough to have a positive male figure in their homes. In addition to this, my father was also a disciplinarian. By today's standards, it may be considered abuse, but when we got out of line, my father corrected that behavior — whether it was by belt, switch, or fist, if necessary. People may disagree with his methods, but none of his children ever spent any time in the custody of the police, which is something not every family in our town could say. I haven't carried my dad's form of discipline into my home, but it worked for us and was not abnormal during the time I was a child. One of the many things I am proud to have learned from my father was the love of my country with all of its promise and its faults. My father taught me to stand, remove my hat, and place my right hand over my heart during the playing of "The Star-Spangled Banner" or when reciting the "Pledge of Allegiance."

On the other hand, my mother was our true *North Star*, the guiding light for our family that kept us together. My mother was the glue that kept my sisters and brothers connected. Since her passing away, we have grown apart, and some of us rarely speak. Like my father, my mother had southern roots with my maternal grandmother, Rosa Mae Hill, being reared in Rock Hill, South Carolina, and my maternal grandfather Alfred David Woodall being raised in Americus, Georgia. The family of my great grandfather Henry Woodall, aka William Henry Woodall Sr., was enslaved in Americus Georgia before 1870.

While my father was an only child, my mother was the eldest daughter of eight children. My mother's family left South Carolina moving to Philadelphia, Pennsylvania, and later settled in Brooklyn, New York. Unlike my father, my mother completed high school prior to entering the workforce. She spent the majority of her working life as an administrative professional with the federal government. However, my mother's work life is not what I remember the most about her. I've lived the vast majority of my adult life without the benefit of her guidance and direction. In the almost twenty-seven years I had her, she taught me compassion. My mother supported every activity we participated in and did her best to show her support for us by attending every event she could. She instilled a love for education and a desire to be a good parent in me. I've heard countless times that a girl's father is the first man in her life and probably the most influential. I would argue that my mother influenced me more than any other person in my life, and for better or worse, shaped me into the man I have become today. She provided balance to the disciplinarian my father was. My mother taught me how to love unconditionally as well as the importance of family. I vividly recall gathering for dinner with my cousins, aunts, and uncles at my grandmother's home in Crown Heights, Brooklyn, after church for Sunday dinner.

My mother instilled the love for God in all of us. As a child, if we did not attend church, we don't leave the house. Missing church meant no television, no phone, and no hanging with friends. Looking back, my mother's consequences for not attending church wasn't a punishment at all. She reminded us that anything we had no matter how small was a result of God's favor. When my obituary is written, and it says *I found God at an early age*, it will be because of my mother. The lessons regarding the love of family and character I learned from my mother. The positive things I learned from my parents are things that I have attempted to replicate with my daughters. I recall sharing with my cousin's eighteen-year-old daughter about how fortunate she is to have her grandmother in her life. As children, we are taught to obey and honor our parents, but it's not until they are gone that we miss their counsel, hugs, idiosyncrasies, and love. There were nights when prior to my being prescribed mood-stabilizing medications, I would call out to my mother in my sleep wanting nothing more than to be with her in heaven. Memories of seeing my mother on her deathbed were vivid in my dreams, and our last conversation and my feelings of great sorrow when she passed haunted my dreams. In my darkest moments, I sought the comfort of my mother's love and guidance.

Whoever claims to love God yet hates a brother or sister is a liar. For whoever does not love their brother and sister, whom they have seen, cannot love God, whom they have not seen.

- 1 John 4:20 (NIV)

We grew up in a two-parent, largely blue-collar community. The men around us were trash collectors, postal employees, commuter train conductors, and appliance repairmen, to name a few. I only recall one man wearing a suit to work because he worked at a bank. The men in the community were coaches, counselors, and shared father figures for all of us. The other men in the community effectively adopted my one close friend who did not have a father at home, so everyone had a father.

There are those who believe that where a child rests in birth order has a lot to do with their personality. When it comes to my twin sister, I absolutely believe that is the case. It has been said that young siblings are more extroverted as we seek attention from our parents, and may find ourselves in competition with our older sisters and brothers. The need for attention may be a bit exaggerated quality in my twin sister. Within an hour after my being admitted to the hospital, my twin sister, Aretha, made her way to Atlanta from New York City.

She won't like to hear it, but she is the most dramatic one of my siblings. She and I are the youngest two of the eight kids. One could argue that traits attributed to the youngest in birth order theory was true with the two of us; we are both extroverted and don't mind the attention that comes with being the youngest (Dixon, Reyes, Leppert & Pappas (2008).

She routinely attempts to exert herself in what she clearly believes is a void that was left as a result of our late mother. I find myself reminding her that I am grown and don't need a mother figure replacement. There are a lot of really positive things to be said about my sister, and we talked about how to approach interactions before she visited, but it seems my advice/direction fell on deaf ears. I was quite ill when she was in town, but from every account, she did not honor boundaries, which added to the stress that others were experiencing and fractured some relationships. It's been suggested that younger siblings are increasingly social when compared to their other sisters or brothers in an attempt to be heard. There were instances where my sister interjected a voice into conversations with the medical professionals, which proved to be more harmful than helpful. Sometimes that causes conflict, so there are times in which I allow her to revel in the feeling that she is running the show.

In childhood, I found myself fighting some of my sister's battles. She felt empowered to talk trash, knowing she had so many big brothers. Now, as adults, there have been times when our battles have led to periods of time when we didn't communicate, but in the end, we always find our way back to each other. While she was here, she was incredibly helpful — taking some pressure off the family and just being here for us. She did learn how independent my girls are and how they have been taught to fend for themselves, which seemed to confuse her. There were also times when she forgot that there was a woman in the house that I normally allowed to manage everything, but in this instance, I was in no shape to do so. Thankfully, our sister-in-law was around to intervene. My sister's presence was a gift that I will always cherish. Sometimes being there is enough. I was really happy that my twin was partly here during this time because I needed her, but it is also important that she knows she is needed, appreciated, and that I love her. My sister is absolutely a valuable part of my family and support system.

My brother Al and his wife Carrol came up from Florida to see me. I know it was not convenient, and it likely created a financial strain for him, but they came. They were at the hospital every day and were strong for me, and that gave me space to be weak. I was able to show my emotional vulnerability when my body was broken. I learned how to pray when I was in the hospital, and having their support allowed me to do that even much better. I let God in a way that I had never done before because I did not have to display the façade that I had it all together. We have always been close, as close as someone with a seven-year age difference will be. As we became adults, the age difference didn't seem to mean as much. I have watched how he has embraced his blended family and how he interacts with his kids and grandkids. Hopefully, I will one day have the same kind of relationship with my kids, and their kids, like my brother has with his.

I have not spoken to one of my elder brothers and my eldest sister since our aunt's funeral just weeks before I fell ill. I wonder if its coincidence or divine intervention that they have the same birthdate just three years apart. Neither of them came to see me during the period when I was closest to death. I can tell myself that this doesn't bother me, but I would be lying to myself. My brother Andrew is five years my elder, and the both of us always seemed to be in competition. For me, it really seemed to manifest itself in high school athletics. We both played football and ran track. We played different positions; he was a running back, and I was a receiver, but we both were sprinters. We ended up attending different high schools, yet the push was for me to earn more accolades and medals — first place medals in particular. What I never shared with anyone was that the push to excel was not out of competition at all. I looked up to my big brother, and he was the measuring stick I used for success. He protected my sister and me from our abusive father. I learned how to be a protector from the example he set, and he was the metric that I used as a father. While we live some 800 miles away from each other, I watched how he interacts with his sons and hope that I am doing the same for my daughters.

From the earliest memories, I remember my older sister having her own ups and downs. She is eight years my elder, and in a lot of ways we grew up in different homes. While living in the same home provided us with a shared environment, the differences in our ages created non-shared experiences. At the end of the day, I needed to see her when I thought I was going to take my last breath. I needed her when my heart was failing, and when I asked her why she didn't come to see me, she said it was because she didn't have the money with which she could fund the trip. That hurt to hear and is something I don't know if I will ever forgive; the resources to fly her down were always available if she had let it be known that the need was there. That explanation might have been plausible, but I never received a call from her to see how I was doing. That was an excuse I don't think I will ever accept. However, as we are taught in the book of Matthew, "...if you do not forgive others their sins, your Father will not forgive your sins" (6:15 NIV). If I am going to be the man I hope to be, I have to cancel any real or perceived duty I believe my sister owed me. At this moment, I am not ready to do that, but I will pray for God's guidance and strength to get to this place. It is my desire to hand out the mercy that I would like to receive.

I met my brother Mark for the first time when I was twenty-three years old. As I got to know him, I loved him because he's well-mannered and well-cultured. Mark spends his days in the hotel service industry and as an actor. Mark and I have not spoken in person since my surgery, but he's called me a number of times, and we have communicated through text messages. I'm looking forward to seeing Mark when it's safe for either of us to travel. My Brothers Gregory and Kenneth, passed away,

Dr. Arthur D. Vaughn

and I have no doubt that we will see them both one day when we are reunited in heaven.

During the initial months of my illness, surgery, and recovery, my brothers and sisters have meant the world to me. We talked regularly, and I pray for them as they pray for me. Our common bond — rooted in the love our mother — covered us, and the foundation of Christ she instilled in us is a comfort to me in times of need.

20.

"So in Christ we, though many, form one body, and each member belongs to all the others."

- Romans 12:5 (NIV)

F amily and friends comprise the most basic unit of any society. In the year after my heart transplant, I've watched families of blood and families of choice woven into the fabric of my long-term health and support. I don't recall doing this, but apparently, while waiting at the doctor's office, I began contacting people and sharing with them that my heart was failing. I was fortunate to have friends from various walks of my life support my family and me through the transplant journey. There were people who would come and sit with me, read with me, and talk with me. There were those who would simply be present and let me talk excessively or just make me laugh. It is amazing to watch what academics call social capital go into action without anyone asking them to. These social networks ranges from friends from elementary school through graduate school, membership organizations, church members, and friends I've made through this journey called life. A dear friend shared with me that the outpouring of support, "Is a testimony to how I've lived my life and treated others; it is a testament of how people feel about my family."

Simply put, social capital includes the relationships and networks where there is mutual trust and support. (Cervellati & Sunde, 2005). These connections include those who live next door and around the corner, those who offer spiritual, moral, financial, and physical support in times of need (Vaughn, 2015). Examples of the groups and institutions in my case would be my church, boards of directors that I am affiliated with, the various membership organizations I belong to, while the informal groups would be friends and other undefined but important social networks that I have developed over the years. The "groups" that make up social capital are often triggered without being asked to do so. In my case, these groups began to provide support in terms of prayer warriors, financial support, food, a place to stay when family members came to town — even home repairs to ensure that everything would be functional when I came home.

There is a group of men I play golf with weekly who immediately came to see me in the hospital. Those early days in the intensive care unit remained a bit of blur, but I remember Rickie, Nat, Eric, Antwan, and Jacques coming to see me. We would laugh and talk about which course we were going to play next. At the time, neither did they nor I knew how ill I really was. I met these men hanging out at WiseAsh Cigars, a local spot that has come to be considered the clubhouse for a group of us. We spent a significant amount of time there watching football, playing cards, dominos, and of course, bonding over cigars. I recall Andrew, my dear friend, who I met from my time on the advisory board for Trust Bank coming to see me. I won't attempt to name all of the people who came by at the risk of not remembering someone.

While it may seem that support during times of need is routine, my hospital stay reaffirmed that it is not the case for many. We had the privilege of meeting so many people who also had family members who were also waiting for some form of transplant. Unfortunately, many were experiencing one form of major challenge or another. We met families who had to make the choice between a meal or a hotel room because they lacked the money to pay for both. We met families who were struggling because they could not be away from work for fear of losing their job. These are real challenges for so many American families in this income insecure world. Despite the United States being such a wealthy nation, three out of four households in America live on paycheck to paycheck. I would argue that a four-bedroom home in the suburbs with two cars in the garage and less than one thousand dollars in the bank is one of the additional examples of poverty. Some say these families are on the brink of losing it all if one family member loses their job.

In this age of Coronavirus, we see financial instability impacting so many homes. This is not to discount those who live in poverty daily, but serves as a reminder of how many of us are a check away for ruin. When you add the cost of a family member suffering a major illness, income instability becomes intensified.

Jesus replied, "They do not need to go away. You give them something to eat." "We have here only five loaves of bread and

two fish," they answered. "Bring them here to me," he said. And he directed the people to sit down on the grass. Taking the five loaves and the two fish and looking up to heaven, he gave thanks and broke the loaves. Then he gave them to the disciples, and the disciples gave them to the people. They all ate and were satisfied, and the disciples picked up twelve basketfuls of broken pieces that were left over. The number of those who ate was about five thousand men, besides women and children.

- Matthew 14:16-21 (NIV)

Each of my nights in the hospital, my friends and loved ones had meals delivered to the hospital and to our home, often more than we could consume. Many of us don't know what food insecurity feels like. However, the U.S. Department of Agriculture reports that eleven percent of Americans, including eleven million minors, don't have adequate financial resources to know where their next meal is coming from (USDA). The overwhelming support we were provided gave us the opportunity to share food with countless others and remove that burden from them. This was a small gesture, and I don't expect any of the families to remember our names, but what

173

they will remember is that they didn't have to worry about a meal on multiple evenings. I believed it underscored the fact that people above and below the poverty level can experience food insecurity.

This is a complex issue where varying social determinants of health, like housing affordability, low wages, ongoing or sudden health issues coupled with the high cost of healthcare, contributed to households not having the ability to provide adequate food for their families. As a result of the support we received from God in the form of our family and friends, our food stores were multiplied, allowing some of the burden others had on them to be removed. This experience brought home the meaning of the proverb, "There, but for the grace of God, go I." This humbling experience should remind all of us that there are outside factors, such as God's kindness and other factors beyond our control, which plays a huge role in our success in life. How we repay that blessing is important, and for me, it's living a life of service to others.

I experienced a surprise like none I could have ever expected. My employer informed me on my first morning back to the office that due to budget cuts, my services were no longer needed. I was at a loss for words, but I should not have been surprised. This same employer, a well-known local institution of higher education whose focus is to train African American men, neglected to send a get-well card or flowers after my initial diagnosis and surgery. This was a stark contrast to a story I read where another local employer, a major worldwide air carrier, rallied in support of an employee who received a transplant a short time after me. Two African American men found themselves in dire need of a heart transplant: One became ill in a short period of time while the other had been in heart failure for several years. Both held leadership roles at the respective employers. One is a father of four, and the other a father of three.

I was considered "The Miracle Patient" as I was on the waitlist for a very short time (four days) prior to getting a heart, and my initial recovery far exceeded the desired expectations. I would argue that the other gentleman was also a miracle patient, not because of the time he waited for a heart, several years, but because he was notified that a heart was available to him at 3:00 a.m. on Christmas morning. What a better day to learn that you are getting a second chance at life then on the day we celebrate the birth of our savior? I spoke with the recipient via social media; he shared that he couldn't elaborate enough on how awesome the air carrier had been to his family and to him! From the CEO to the 80,000 employees — the prayers, visits to the ICU, donations, and words of encouragement — "My company was there! They also continued to be there as I recover," he exclaimed. We remain in touch and I am thrilled to report that he remains in great health.

We often think of small institutions of higher education as insular organizations that display characteristics of a family. These organizations operate inside of a bit of a bubble with close-knit ties to one another. Shockingly, the current leadership of this institution seems to be out of step with their employees: their lives, their wants, and their needs. I elected not to dwell on what, in my estimation, was a lack of character and empathy by a small number of people and left it for the lawyers to address. The institution is one that I have great respect for, and serving there was a career goal. If it is in God's plan, I will one day return under different leadership and make the contribution I had hoped.

I turned to address more immediate needs. I had just gone through a $1.4 million-dollar surgery that left a co-payment of $276,000 along with a monthly bill of $7,698 for ongoing treatment, not including the cost to fill the prescriptions for the life-saving pills I took on a daily. I've never shared that cost of the procedure with my family, as I would prefer that my family not be burdened with this information. I will work through the cost of the surgery. The anxiety and stress of this mounting debt have become so overwhelming that I am sure my disposition and attitude was challenged. I turned to prayer, but soon after, despair took over. There was a time when I was angry with my employer at the time; however, as I have grown in Christ, "I have forgiven them, as you asked." (Numbers 14:20 NIV).

"And my God will meet all your needs according to the riches of his glory in Christ Jesus."

- Philippians 4:19 (NIV)

I thought I had already experienced the lowest point in my life, but I experienced a new low. I was going to have to look my daughter in the eyes and tell her that I couldn't provide for her. As a father, a man, and self-proclaimed #GirlDad, I simply couldn't believe it had come to this. She was enrolled in college and had an outstanding bill for the spring term. Over the last seven months I depleted my savings account, my medical bills are beginning to pile up, and I had been told that due to budget cuts I would not be returning to work after a heart transplant.

Not long before, I was in a position to help others, and I did. Now that I am in need of help, I am ashamed and embarrassed. It may be a male ego thing, but I didn't want to ask others for help. There was a time I would have gone and gotten any odd job I could; pushing grocery carts or mopping floors to get what's needed with having multiple degrees be damned. But today, I am not physically able to do the things I would have done in the past. My level of anxiety and stress was at an all-time high. I wasn't thinking about this unplanned procedure and the associated cost. I wasn't thinking about what I termed a heartless employer. I was thinking, how did I let things get to this point? How did I let things get so out of control?

In retrospect, what was truly happening was that my faith was being tested. I believe God gives us tools to handle any situation, and if we have faith in Him, He will definitely make a way. The masculine template suggests that we take care of our families, whatever it takes. The challenge is "whatever it takes" often does not include asking others for help when we need it. Many of us find it incredibly difficult and humbling to ask for help, even a bit embarrassing. In this case, "Man Up" needs to mean being humble enough to ask for help.

That day, I found myself doing what I previously thought

was unthinkable; I sent a message out to a group of friends, some closer than others. The message explained my situation and asked each of them for a small loan. I am hoping that this will allow me to pay my daughter's tuition, and when I get back to work, I can pay them all back. Typing the note was an emotional moment and a humbling experience. Outwardly, I portray this guy that has it all and is under control. In reality, I am just trying to hold it all together. I turned to my faith — that if I prayed, God would show me a path to my destination. The same reluctance that prevents men from asking for help is the same "be a man" approach that leads us to not listen to our bodies when something is wrong. It's the same misconceived notion of manhood that is contributing to our premature deaths.

I couldn't tell this story without sharing the outcome. My friends stepped up and helped me out. I asked a small group for help, and I paid the balance due on my daughter's tuition. My sense was that if I had asked others, more would have been given. God gave me the names, and they helped me. I will now repay that unmerited favor with acts of service.

"Worship the Lord your God, and his blessing will be on your food and water. I will take away sickness from among you."

- Exodus 23:25 (NIV)

Dr. Arthur D. Vaughn

Throughout the fall of 2019, my body's immune system was rejecting my new heart. In early 2020 it felt like we were beginning to turn the corner and get this illness under control, and along came COVID-19 (Corona Virus). I was social distancing since August 2019 and before COVID-19 got its name. I thought I was going to be able to begin working again and return to a modified level of socializing with friends and family, only to be told that I needed to extend the self-quarantine. I began this self-hibernation five months earlier due to my being at high risk because of my transplant surgery. This new severe intense respiratory condition was first discovered in China in December 2019 and grew to become a global pandemic (coronavirus.gov). The world had not experienced anything like this in my lifetime. While I was already self-quarantined and social distancing, I was now being joined in this effort by most of the world. We saw schools closing, businesses either closing or having their employees work from home, and unemployment reach heights that had not been seen since the Great Depression. The Centers for Disease Control and Prevention suggests that the COVID-19 symptoms closely resemble those of the flu with fever & respiratory distress. (coronavirus.gov). According to *The Journal of Heart and Lung*

Transplantation

Doctors Aslam & Mehra argued that transplant patients are at greater risk of contracting COVID-19 because of our weaker immune systems, and the treatment to address the illness added to the risk we face. As recipients, we also had to consider how the management for Coronavirus increases our risk. The treatment includes discontinuation of the drugs used to suppress the transplant patient's immune systems as well as introducing new antibodies while treating the patient with high doses of anti-inflammatory drugs. This treatment is particularly risky for transplant patients because we take drugs to prevent our immune system from attacking the new organ that was placed in our body, and the treatment for COVID-19 does the exact opposite of the treatment we needed in order to survive. Transplant patients have to be more diligent than the general population when social distancing, practicing hand hygiene, and be even more careful to avoid potentially infected individuals.

21.

"I have told you these things, so that in me you may have peace. In this world you will have trouble. But take heart! I have overcome the world."

- John 16:33 (NIV)

During quiet moments, I find myself being still and thinking about all that happened last summer; it regularly overwhelms me and causes worry that it will happen again. It makes me anxious, as the ordeal was the most extreme experience I've ever had, and stills scares me to this day. I'm not sure anyone is ever prepared for major trauma, but this rocked my world, and as much as I pretended, I have not made peace with it.

I try to keep my experience in perspective; I am not the first or last to receive a heart transplant. But I'm hoping my story can be an inspiration to someone — a source of comfort to someone who thinks all is lost. Less than a year after my operation, the Georgia Transplant Foundation asked me to consider becoming a mentor to future patients and families going through the process.

Attempting to become useful again is proving to be more difficult than I ever expected. I am seeking tools to address the episodes I am having. Today, I began to wonder if my mind is becoming fragile from a lack of use. I was used to solving problems and equations for ten or more hours per day. Now, interaction has been limited. So, I'm endeavoring to engage in conversations with other people, as it's just starting to click for me that my resting mind may be a contributing factor to the episodes. I would interact and lead people and projects, and interact with people during all of my waking hours. It is time for me to take the next step in my healing process.

Recently, the team tasked with my rehabilitation suggested to volunteer with a nonprofit as both is an act of service as well as a mental health coping strategy. I am going to commit to adjusting my eating habits, so that I can get to a healthy weight. I am going to commit to continued therapy and address issues that continue to haunt me. Going forward, I have to focus on my physical, mental, and financial health. We have to redefine "Manhood" and what it means to "Man Up." What better way to "Man Up" than to make sure that you go in for an annual physical during your birth month. What better show of manhood is there than to make sure you are listening to your body and taking care of yourself so you can be there for those you love and who love you?

22.

Very truly I tell you, unless a kernel of wheat falls to the ground and dies, it remains only a single seed. But if it dies, it produces many seeds. Anyone who loves their life will lose it, while anyone who hates their life in this world will keep it for eternal life. Whoever serves me must follow me; and where I am, my servant also will be. My Father will honor the one who serves me.

- John 12:24-26 (NIV)

My therapist, Dr. Parkins has a Mark Twain quote tattooed on her arm that reads, "That the two most important days in your life are the day you are born and the day you find out why!"

I was born on March 14, 1969

I found out why on August 24, 2019

August 24th was the day I woke up to God's glory! I woke up yelling, "I Need Help! I Need Help!" I believe what I was really saying is "I Need God! I Need God!" Through the Holy Spirit, my surgeons were able to give me a new heart and a second chance at life. But what I did not know was what God's plan was for me. I knew I felt sorrowful because someone else had to die that I may live, but is that not the same story of Jesus Christ? The Bible teaches us in John 12:24-26 that Jesus told His disciples that he was going to die, but through His death, we would live. Surely, I am not saying that I am Christ, but I am saying I needed and continue to need God. God loved me when I did not love myself. It was revealed to me through this ordeal that I was not living a life that would be pleasing in the eyes of God, and He was not only giving me a chance to change, but He also was giving me the opportunity to be a blessing to others.

Not long after my transplant, I heard from someone whom I had met through my walk in life whose spouse was on the heart transplant list at the same hospital. Her husband of many years had been on the waitlist of a transplant for a long time. Unfortunately, you have to go through various stages of illness before you are moved to the top of this list. The gentleman is an introvert and wasn't comfortable talking about his feelings. But as someone who had just gone through the process, I knew what he was feeling. I knew what it was like to sit alone in the quiet times and pray for healing. I also knew what the wait does to you mentally. We were able to talk, and I was able to share with him that there is hope. We can see the impact heart failure has on our body, but the impact on our mind is hidden from view. You can recover physically, but you can also recover from the unspoken toll this illness takes on your mental state. Through this process, I learned how to pray for him as others had prayed for me.

Normally, hospital day for me was Thursday, but due to scheduling conflicts, I went earlier in the week on this occasion. I had not spoken to the family who was waiting on the heart for a while. On this morning, not only did I see them, I discovered that he was back for his first follow up appointment after being blessed with a new heart, "Won't He do it! There is power in the name of Jesus!" I learned a great deal about resilience and the healing power of prayer. Later that day I received a text from the spouse of the gentleman I spoke to, "He really enjoyed talking with you. Thanks so much, it was super encouraging."

On July 19, 2019, I was placed on the top of the transplant

list. On July 20, 2020, I officially became a mentor with the Georgia Transplant Foundation. Through my first year of healing, I have told my story countless times in multiple places. There have been instances when people have let me know that my experience has had a positive impact on their life. You never know how much you are impacting others with your words. My openness about my post-traumatic stress has led to my friend, Kevin, talking openly about the mental health challenges he was experiencing after he had life-saving surgery. That is what this book is about, letting people know that they are not alone. You can experience remorse and talk about it. Letting people know it is okay not to be okay, and that there is help for them.

We have to Man Up and listen to our bodies! We have to Man Up and see our primary care physicians annually. We have to Man Up and acknowledge that we may suffer from short-term or long-term mental health issues. We have to Man Up and seek help from God in the form of a therapist! We have to Man Up and talk about our individual challenges! We have to Man Up!

Appendix

1. Barnes, V., Schneider, R., Alexander, C., & Staggers, F. (1997). Stress, stress reduction, and hypertension in African Americans: an updated review. *Journal of the National Medical Association, 89*(7), 464.

2. Beer, J., & Horn, J. (2000). The influence of rearing order on personality development within two adoption cohorts. Journal of Personality, 68, 789–819.

3. Bible, H. (1984). New International Version (NIV). *Grand Rapids: Zondervan.*

4. Cervellati, M., & Sunde, U. (2005). Human capital formation, life expectancy, and the process of development. *American Economic Review, 95*(5), 1653-1672.

5. Chung, M. L., Pressler, S. J., Dunbar, S. B., Lennie, T. A., Moser, D. K., & Endowed, G. (2010). Predictors of depressive symptoms in caregivers of patients with heart failure. *The Journal of cardiovascular nursing, 25*(5), 411.

6. Dixon, M. M., Reyes, C. J., Leppert, M. F., & Pappas, L. M. (2008). Personality and birth order in large families. *Personality and individual differences*, 44(1), 119-128.

7. Galdas PM, Cheater F, Marshall P. Men and health help-seeking behavior: literature review. J Adv Nursing. 2005 Mar;49(6):616–23.   http://dx.doi.org/10.1111   /j.1365-2648.2004.03331.x

8. Hankerson, S. H., Fenton, M. C., Geier, T. J., Keyes, K. M., Weissman, M. M., & Hasin, D. S. (2011). Racial differences in symptoms, comorbidity, and treatment for major depressive disorder among black and white adults. Journal of the National Medical Association, 103(7), 576-584

9. Hankerson, S. H., Suite, D., & Bailey, R. K. (2015). Treatment disparities among African American men with depression: Implications for clinical practice. Journal of health care for the poor and underserved, 26(1), 21.

10. Hasin DS, Goodwin RD, Stinson FS, et al. Epidemiology

of major depressive disorder: results from the National Epidemiologic Survey on Alcoholism and Related Conditions. Arch Gen Psychiatry. 2005 Oct;62(10):1097–106. http://dx.doi.org/10.1001/arch psyc.62.10.1097

11. Holland, B. (2017). The 'Father of Modern Gynecology' Performed Shocking Experiments on Slaves. History Stories.

12. Kübler-Ross, E., & Kessler, D. (2005). On grief and grieving: Finding the meaning of grief through the five stages of loss. Simon and Schuster.

13. Litman, T. J. (1974). The family as a basic unit in health and medical care: A social-behavioral overview. Social Science & Medicine (1967), 8(9-10), 495-519.

14. https://www.mayoclinic.org/diseases-conditions/anaphylaxis/symptoms-causes/syc-20351468 https://www.mayoclinic.org/diseases-conditions/anaphylaxis/symptoms-causes/syc-20351468

15. Möller-Leimkühler AM, Bottlender R, Straus A, et al. Is

there evidence for a male depressive syndrome in inpatients with major depression? J Affect Disord. 2004 May;80(1):87–93. http://dx.doi.org/10.1016/S0165-0327(03)00051-X

16. Mota-Pereira, J., Silverio, J., Carvalho, S., Ribeiro, J. C., Fonte, D., & Ramos, J. (2011). Moderate exercise improves depression parameters in treatment-resistant patients with major depressive disorder. Journal of psychiatric research, 45(8), 1005-1011.

17. National Alliance for Caregiving. (2005) *Caregiving in the US*. AARP; Bethesda, MD: The National Alliance for Caregiving.

18. Ojanuga, D. (1993). The medical ethics of the'father of gynaecology', Dr J Marion Sims. Journal of medical ethics, 19(1), 28-31.

19. Oquendo MA, Ellis SP, Greenwald S, et al. Ethnic and sex differences in suicide rates relative to major depression in the United States. Am J Psychiatry. 2001 Oct;158(10):1652–8. http://dx.doi.org/10.1176/appi.ajp.158.10.1652

20. Trivedi Madhukar, H. (2008). Treatment strategies to improve and sustain remission in major depressive disorder. Dialogues in clinical neuroscience, 10(4), 377.

21. United States Department of Agriculture - https://www.ers.usda.gov/

22. Vaughn, A. D. (2015). The Effect of Need-and Merit-based Aid on Degree Attainment at Georgia's Public Colleges and Universities (Doctoral dissertation, University of Georgia).

23. Wilkes, G. (2011). Jesus on leadership: Timeless wisdom on servant leadership. Tyndale House Publishers, Inc.

24. Williams, D. R., Gonzalez, H. M., Neighbors, H., Nesse, R., Abelson, J. M., Sweetman, J., & Jackson, J. S. (2007). Prevalence and distribution of major depressive disorder in African Americans, Caribbean blacks, and non-Hispanic whites: results from the National Survey of American Life. *Archives of general psychiatry, 64*(3), 305-315.

CPSIA information can be obtained
at www.ICGtesting.com
Printed in the USA
LVHW011356301020
670160LV00004B/373